Snooky the Snail's™
Preschool Fluency Worksheets

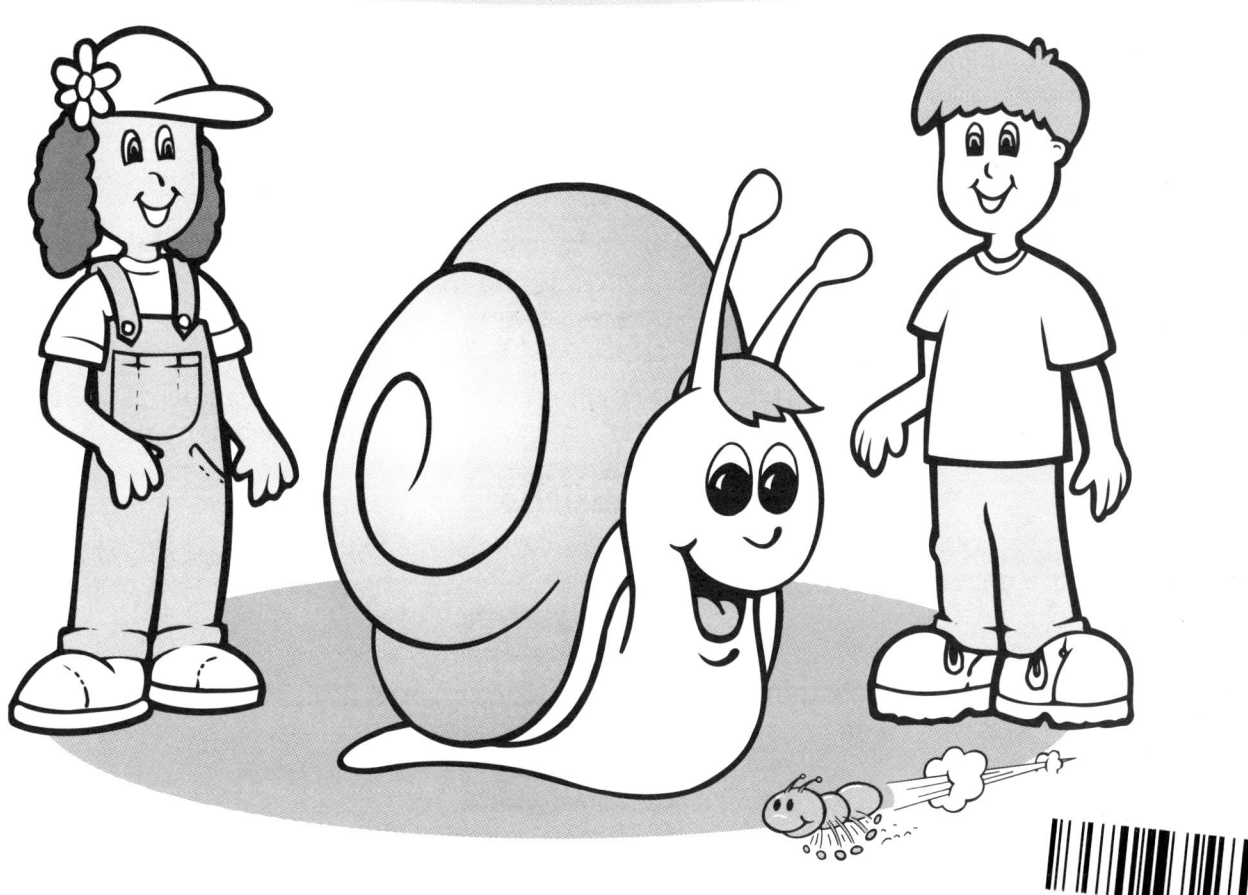

Written by Monica Gustafson
Illustrated by Rick Rowland

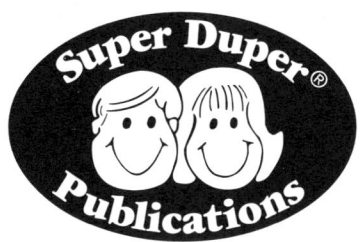

Copyright ©2002, SUPER DUPER® PUBLICATIONS, a division of Super Duper®, Inc. All rights reserved. Permission is granted for the user to reproduce the material contained herein in limited form for classroom use only. Reproduction of this material for an entire school or school system is strictly prohibited. No part of this material may be reproduced (except as noted above), stored in a retrieval system, or transmitted in any form or by any means (mechanically, electronically, recording, web, etc.) without the prior written consent and approval of Super Duper® Publications.

www.superduperinc.com
1-800-277-8737

ISBN# 978-1-58650-057-3

Introduction

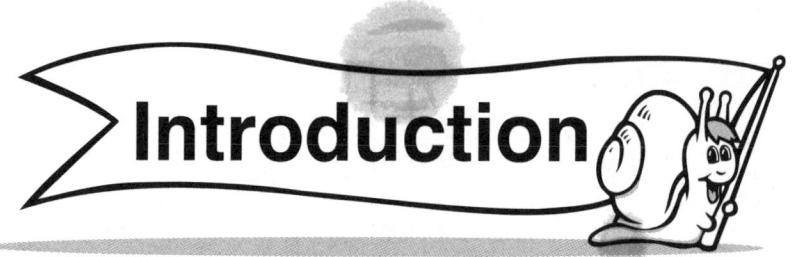

This *Snooky the Snail Preschool Fluency Workbook* is divided into 8 sections of easy-to-use worksheets which can be incorporated into any fluency program or used as structured home programming for parents.

Section 1

In the first section children are introduced to Snooky, a little snail who tries to crawl too fast and bumps himself with his shell. His Mom explains that some people can't do things fast, and if you do things slow and easy you don't feel the "bumps." The children are then encouraged to help Snooky move "slow and easy" through the worksheets. A finger puppet is provided for children to manipulate as they use their slow, easy voices and touch or trace Snooky's trail through the worksheets.

Pictures are provided (in the back of the book) for each of the next four sections. The SLP and child can select the vocabulary for practice from a variety of appropriate pictures. Each picture can be verbally practiced slow and easy as it is cut and pasted in place for later practice ... or for when Snooky makes his way around the page.

Section 2

Single word vocabulary: The child cuts and pastes pictures into a variety of situations (an elephant parade, frog's lily pad, etc.) and then, using a slow and easy voice, names each picture.

Section 3

A ... or a noun and a noun ...: When asked questions like, "What did Snooky see at the farm?" the child will respond with "a horse" or "a horse and a cow." A slow and easy voice is used.

Section 4

I want ...: In this section the child tells Snooky personal preferences such as "I like ..." or "I want ..." A slow and easy voice is used.

Section 5

Increased length sentence utterances: The child answers Snooky's questions using a slow easy voice and increased length utterances such as, "I don't like to eat ..." or "My mom has brown hair."

Section 6

Spontaneous open set fluency: In each scene Snooky explores places like the classroom, farm, or playground. Using a slow and easy voice, the child will describe what is in the scene or what Snooky is doing.

Section 7

Puppets and Scenes for Role-playing!

Section 8

Picture Library

Table of Contents

Section 1 — pages

Let's meet Snooky the Snail! (Story) 1–6
Snooky Finger Puppet 7

Section 2

Snooky likes to travel (See pages 76-92 for vocabulary pictures) 10
Snooky drives a train (See pages 76-92 for vocabulary pictures) 11
Snooky makes friends (See pages 76-92 for vocabulary pictures) 12
Snooky visits the pond (See pages 76-92 for vocabulary pictures) 13
Snooky washes clothes (See pages 76-92 for vocabulary pictures) 14
Snooky goes to the circus (See pages 76-92 for vocabulary pictures) 15
Snooky goes house hunting (See pages 76-92 for vocabulary pictures) 16
Snooky blows speech bubbles (See pages 76-92 for vocabulary pictures) 17
Snooky and Carol Caterpillar (See pages 76-92 for vocabulary pictures) 18

Section 3

Snooky visits your classroom (See page 88 for vocabulary pictures) 20
Snooky visits the zoo (See page 90 for vocabulary pictures) 21
Snooky visits the farm (See page 82 for vocabulary pictures) 22
Family drawing activity (See page 81 for vocabulary pictures) 23
Things that are red (See page 89 for vocabulary pictures) 24
Things that are yellow (See page 89 for vocabulary pictures) 25
Snooky visits the refrigerator (See pages 83-85 for vocabulary pictures) 26
Snooky meets your friends (See page 81 for vocabulary pictures) 27
Snooky decorates the Christmas tree (See page 78 for vocabulary pictures) 28

Section 4

What did you see at school? (See page 88 for vocabulary pictures) 30
What do you like to eat? (See pages 83-85 for vocabulary pictures) 31
What can you do at the playground? (See page 87 for vocabulary pictures) 32
What did you buy when you went shopping? (See pages 83-86 for vocabulary pictures) 33
What is in your toy box? (See page 87 for vocabulary pictures) 34
What do you want for your birthday? (See page 87 for vocabulary pictures) 35
What do you wear when it is hot outside? (See page 80 for vocabulary pictures) 36
What do you wear when it is cold outside? (See page 80 for vocabulary pictures) 37
What did you see at the zoo? (See page 90 for vocabulary pictures) 38

Section 5 pages

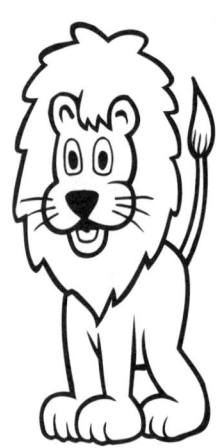

- Draw a picture of your Mom (See page 81 for vocabulary pictures) 40
- Draw a picture of your Dad (See page 81 for vocabulary pictures) 41
- Draw a picture of your bedroom (See page 77 for vocabulary pictures) 42
- Draw a picture of your pet (See pages 82 and 91 for vocabulary pictures) 43
- Draw a picture of your playground (See page 87 for vocabulary pictures) 44
- Draw a picture of something you don't like to eat (See pages 83-85 for vocabulary pictures) 45
- Draw a picture of something you like to wear (See pages 80 for vocabulary pictures) 46
- Draw a picture of what you saw at the circus (See page 79 for vocabulary pictures) 47
- Draw a picture of what you saw at the beach (See page 76 for vocabulary pictures) 48
- Draw a picture of what you saw at the grocery store (See pages 83-86 for vocabulary pictures) 49
- Draw a picture of what you saw at the toy store (See page 87 for vocabulary pictures) 50

Section 6

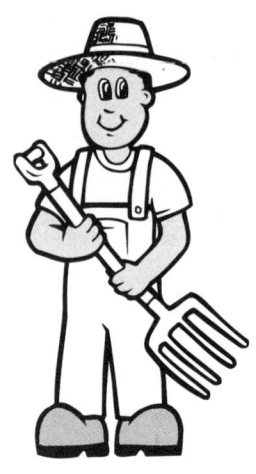

- Search and find Snooky on the farm 52
- Search and find Snooky on the playground 53
- Search and find Snooky at school 54
- Search and find Snooky at the zoo 55
- Search and find Snooky at the birthday party 56
- Search and find Snooky at the beach 57
- Search and find Snooky at the picnic 58
- Search and find Snooky at the Halloween party 59
- Search and find Snooky in the winter scene 60
- Search and find Snooky in the Christmas scene 61
- Search and find Snooky at the Easter egg hunt 62

Section 7

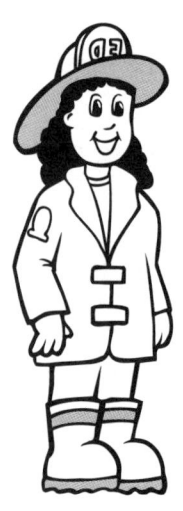

- Instructions on role-playing with puppets and scenes 64
- The Castle 65
- Fantasy Garden 66
- Jungle Scene 67
- Under the Sea 68
- Alien Planet 69
- The Fire Station 70
- At the Circus 71
- Police Officer 72
- On the Farm 73
- The North Pole 74

Section 8

Reproducible Picture Library	76–92
Beach	76
Bedroom	77
Christmas/Easter	78
Circus	79
Clothing	80
Family and Friends	81
Farm Pictures	82
Food	83–85
Grocery Store (Non-food items)	86
Playground/Toys/Birthday	87
School	88
Things that are Red or Yellow	89
Zoo Pictures	90
X-Tra Pictures for Fun!	91
Draw Your Own Pictures	92

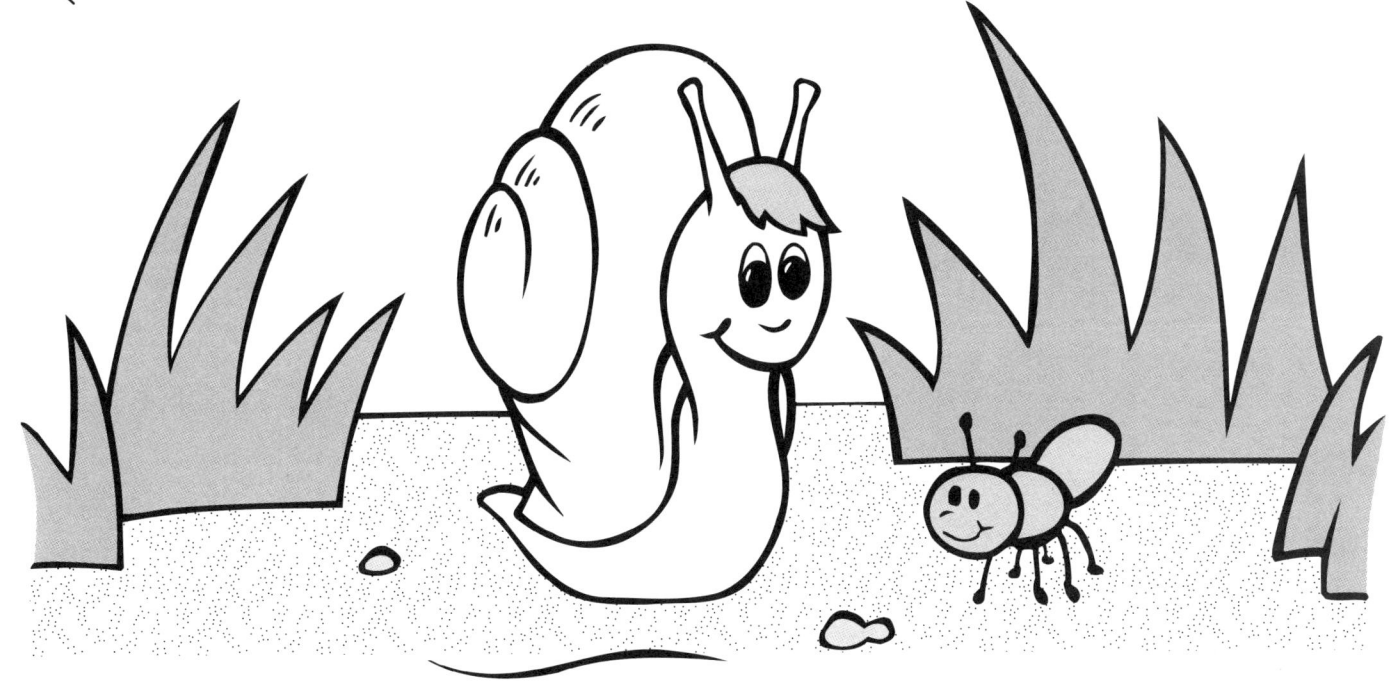

Section 1
Let's meet Snooky the Snail!

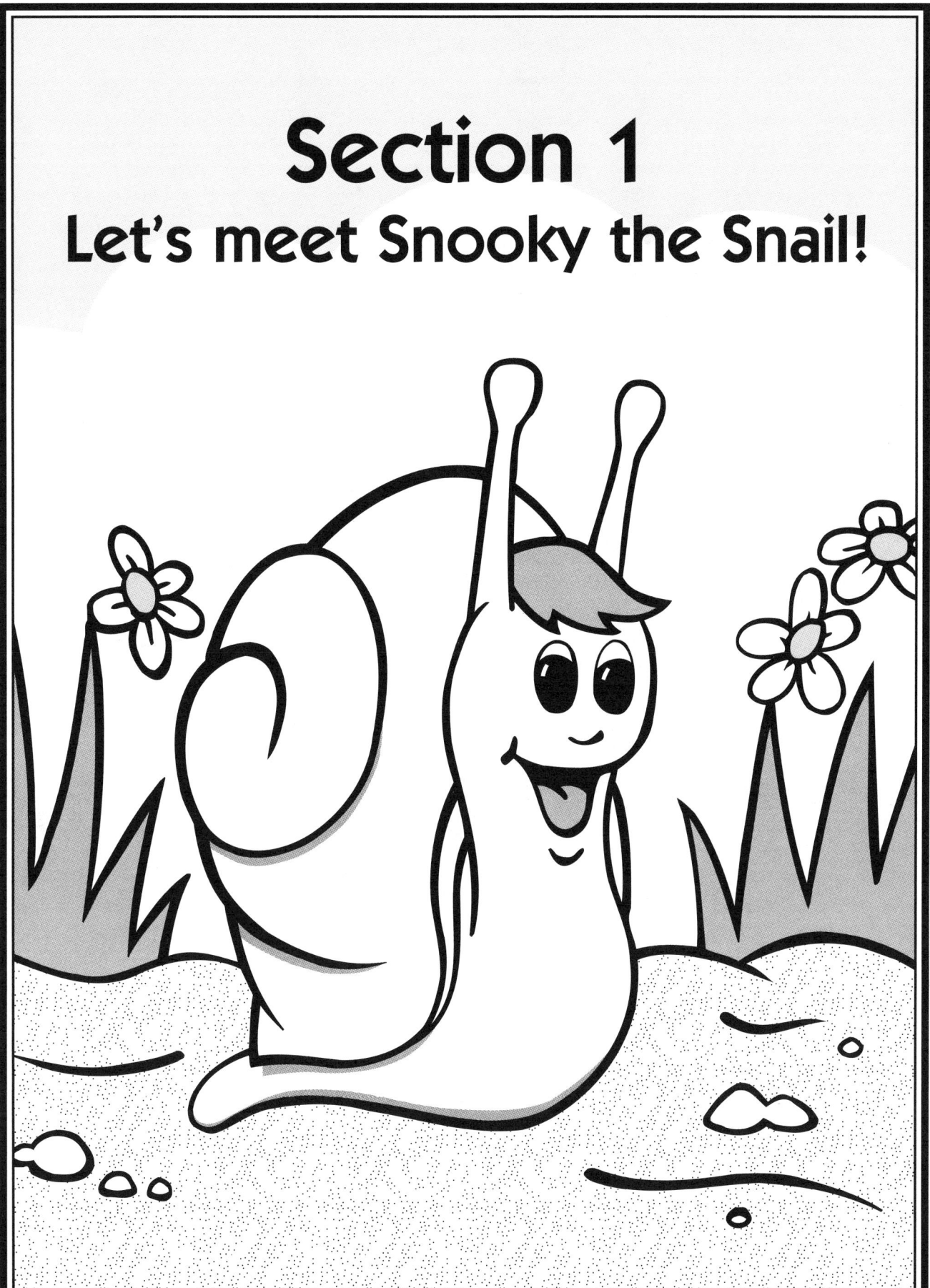

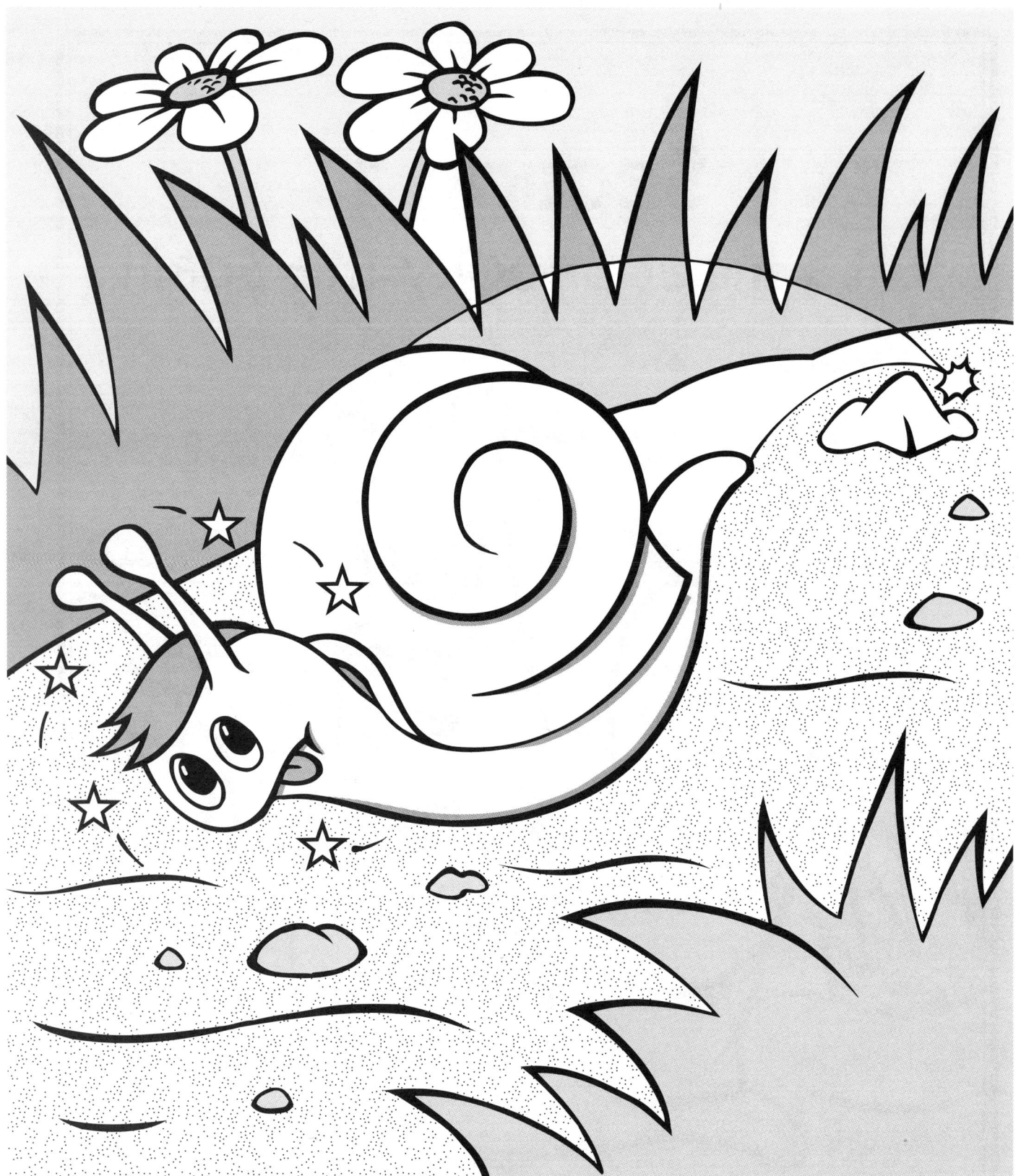

Snooky was a little snail who was always in a hurry. Snooky was in such a hurry all the time that he tripped over everything. And when Snooky tripped, his shell would slide forward and bump him in the back of the head. His Mother tried to tell Snooky that he was going to have to slow down.

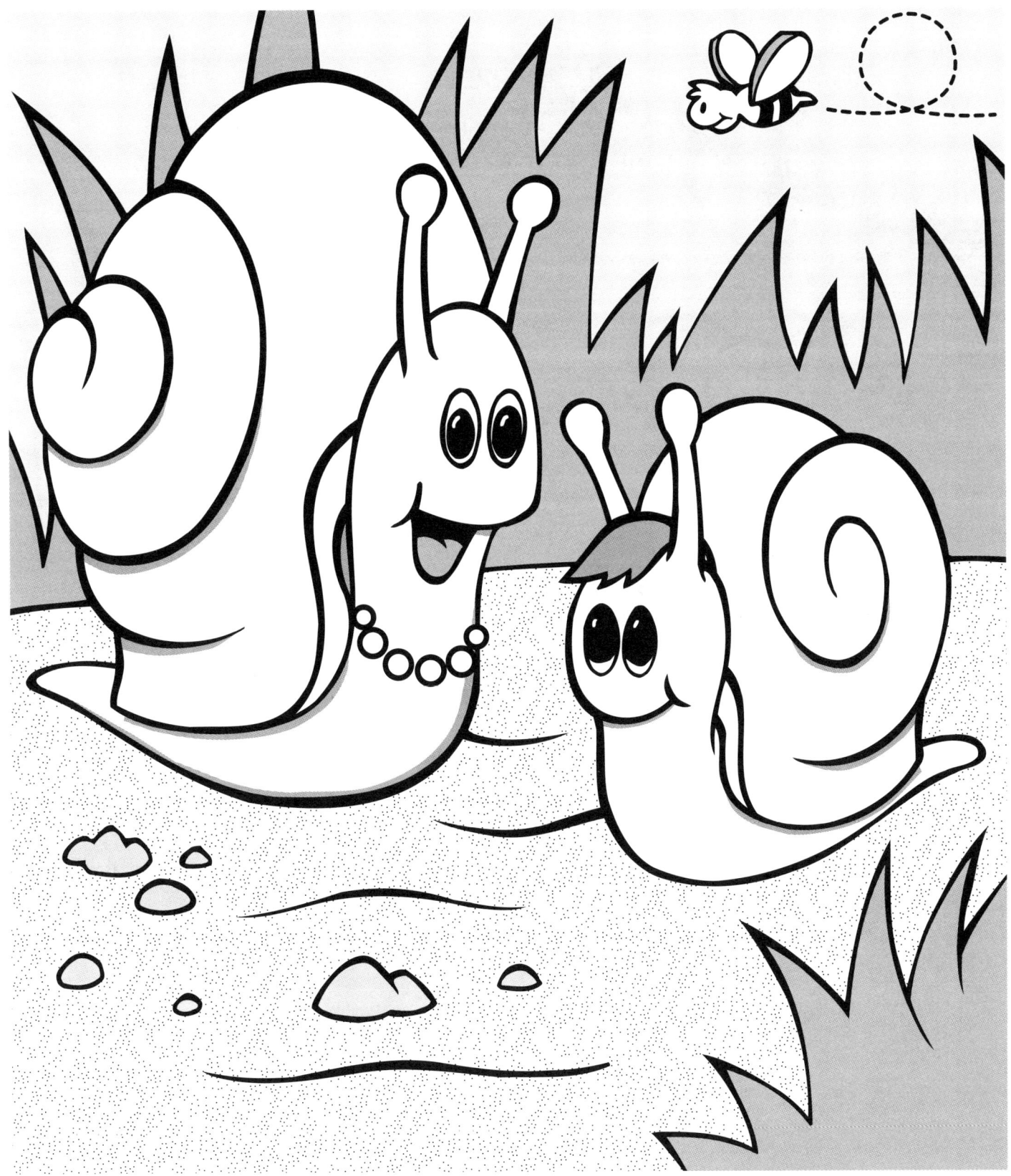

"Snails are not meant to move fast," she said. "Snails move along slowly and smoothly over everything. Even if we are going over a bumpy spot, when we go slow and smooth and easy, it doesn't feel bumpy."

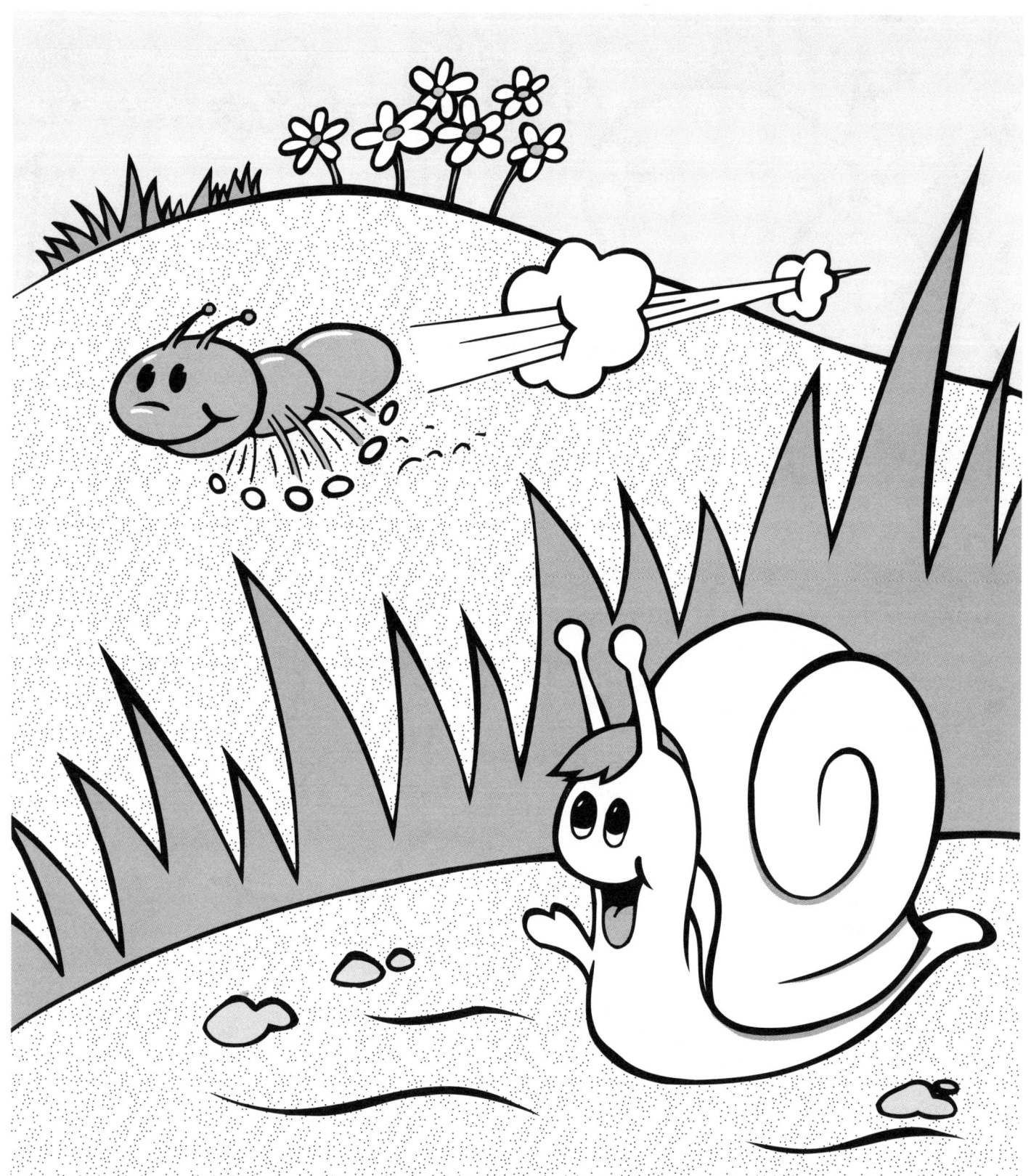

"But I want to move fast," said Snooky. "Why can't I move as fast as an ant?" he asked. "Well," said his Mother, "the ant might be able to move fast, but he can't carry his house on his back like we do," she explained. "Everyone can do something well; the ant moves quickly and we carry our houses with us. That is very special."

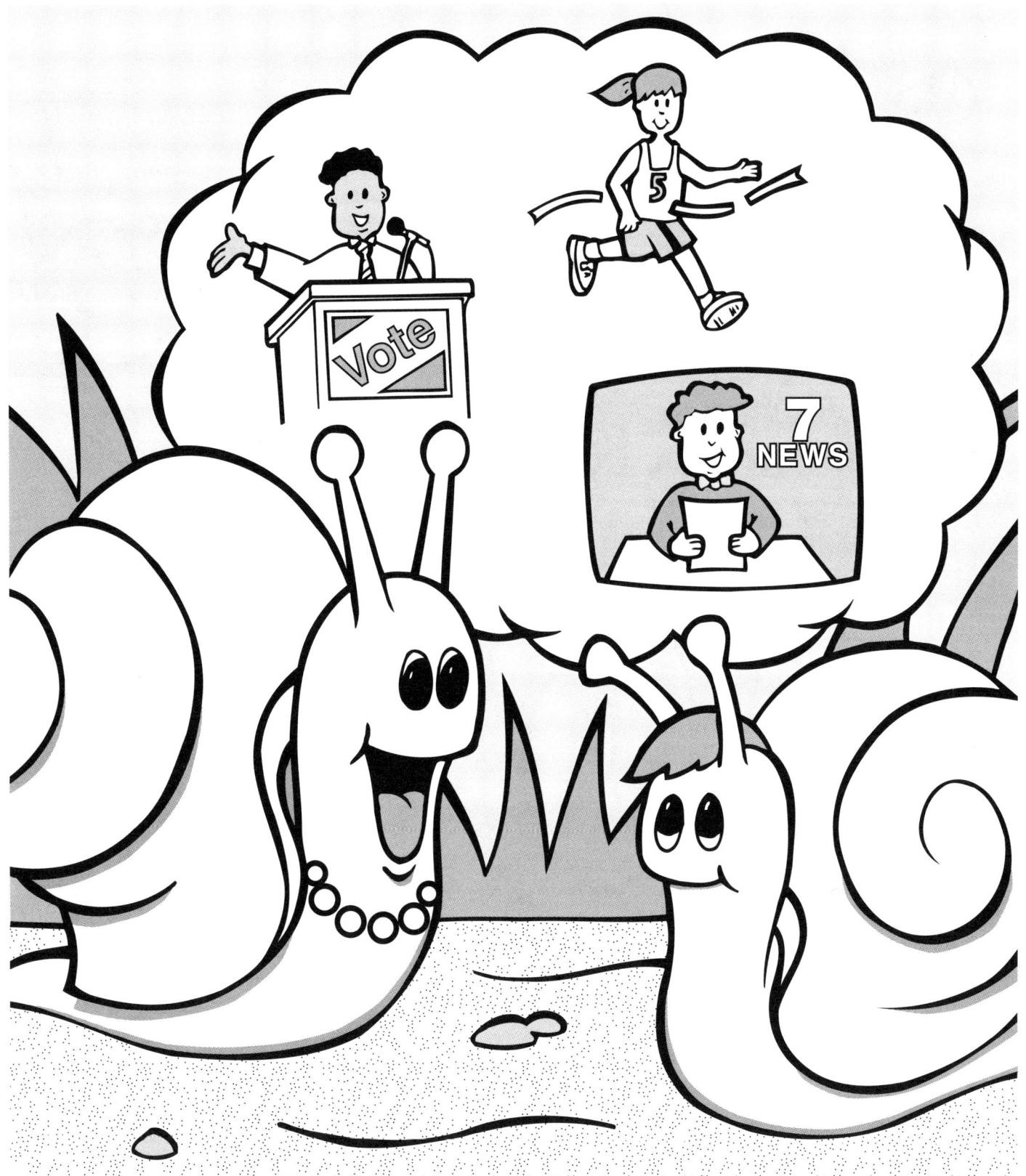

"Even people have special things they can do. Some people can run fast, some people can read fast, and some people can talk fast. But just like us snails, if you can't do something fast, there is nothing wrong with doing it slow. When you do things slow, smooth and easy, you don't feel the bumps."

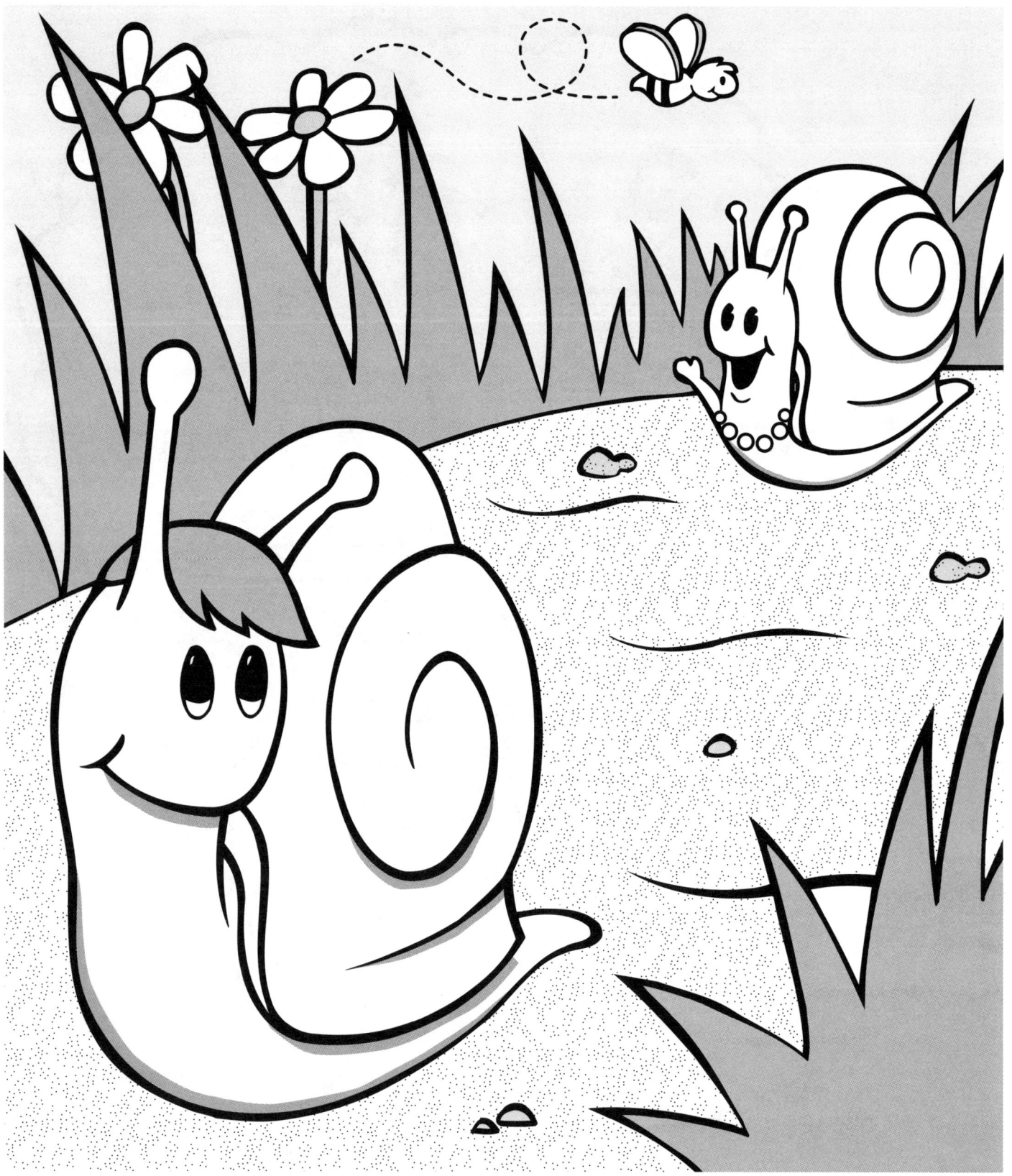

"Okay," said Snooky, "I will try to move slow, smooth and easy. Maybe then everything won't seem so bumpy."

    Let's follow Snooky to make sure he does things slow, smooth and easy. Let's help him do things so they aren't so bumpy.

Snooky Finger Puppet

Copy, color and cut out Snooky. Staple where shown. Insert finger. Now you have a finger puppet!

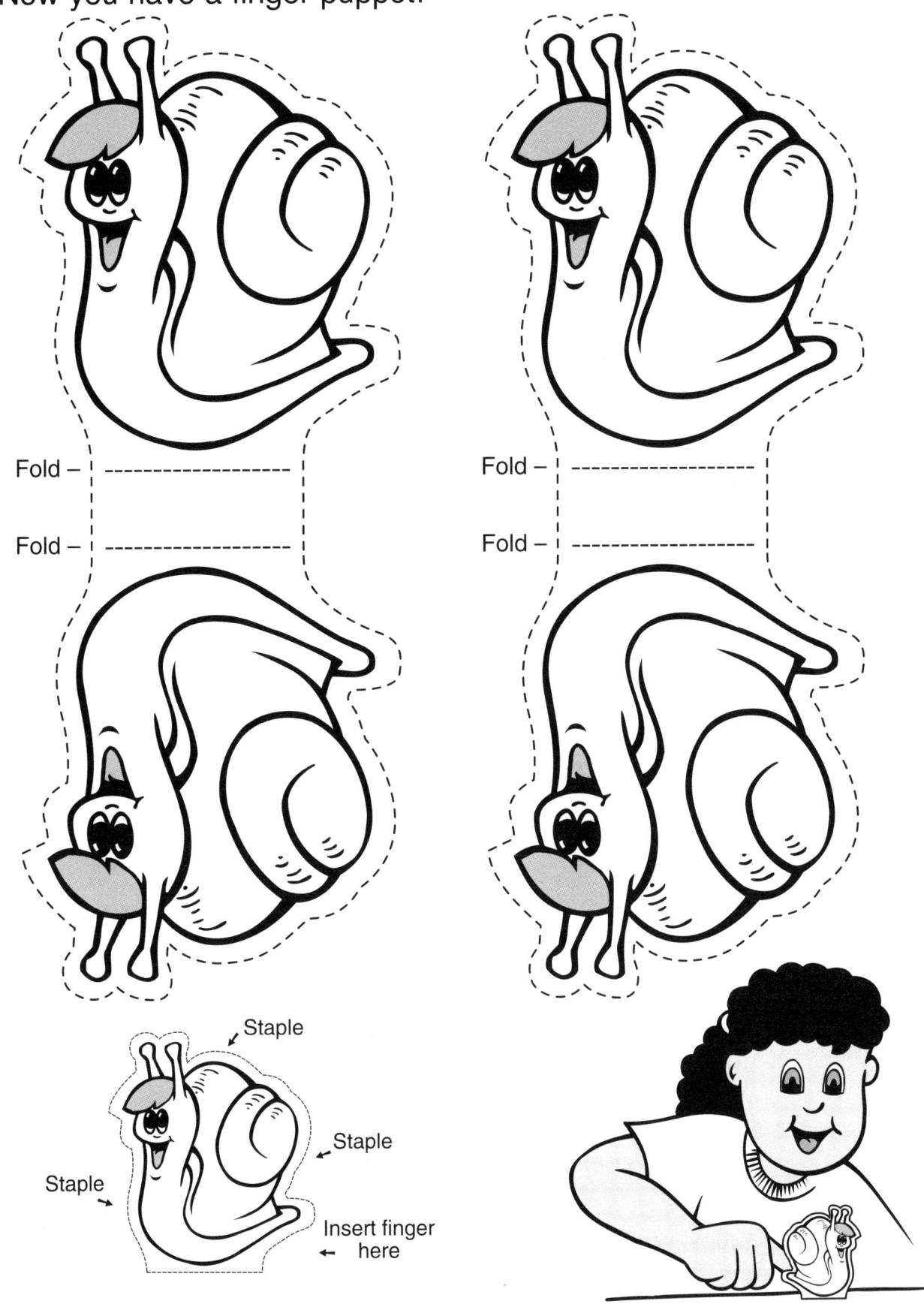

Section 2

Goal: To have child produce single word vocabulary using a slow and easy voice.

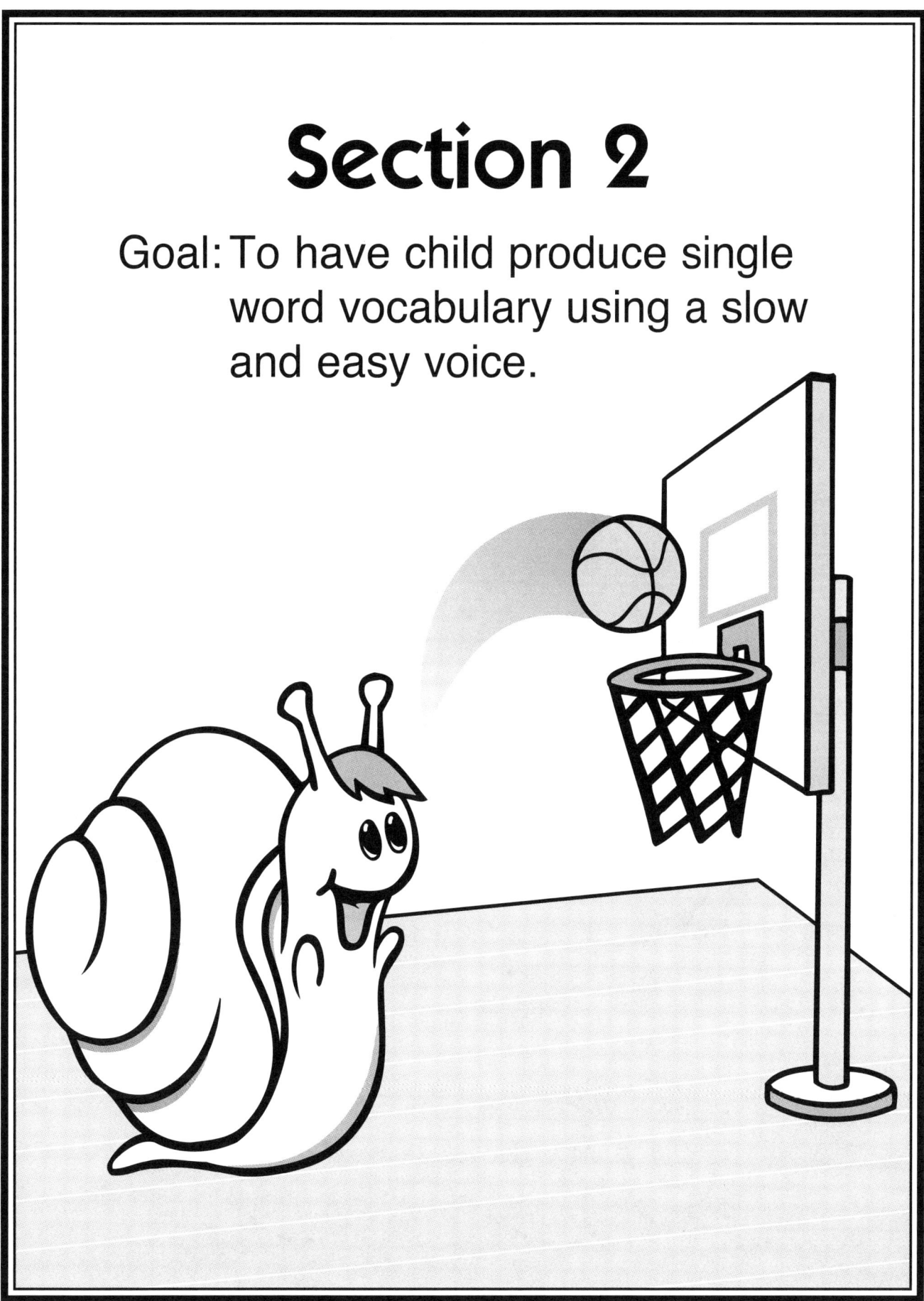

Snooky likes to travel! Color, cut and paste your pictures at the beginning of each hill (see pages 76-92). Make your Snooky finger puppet (see page 7) and trace over the sound hills with it. Use your slow and easy voice as you say each word.

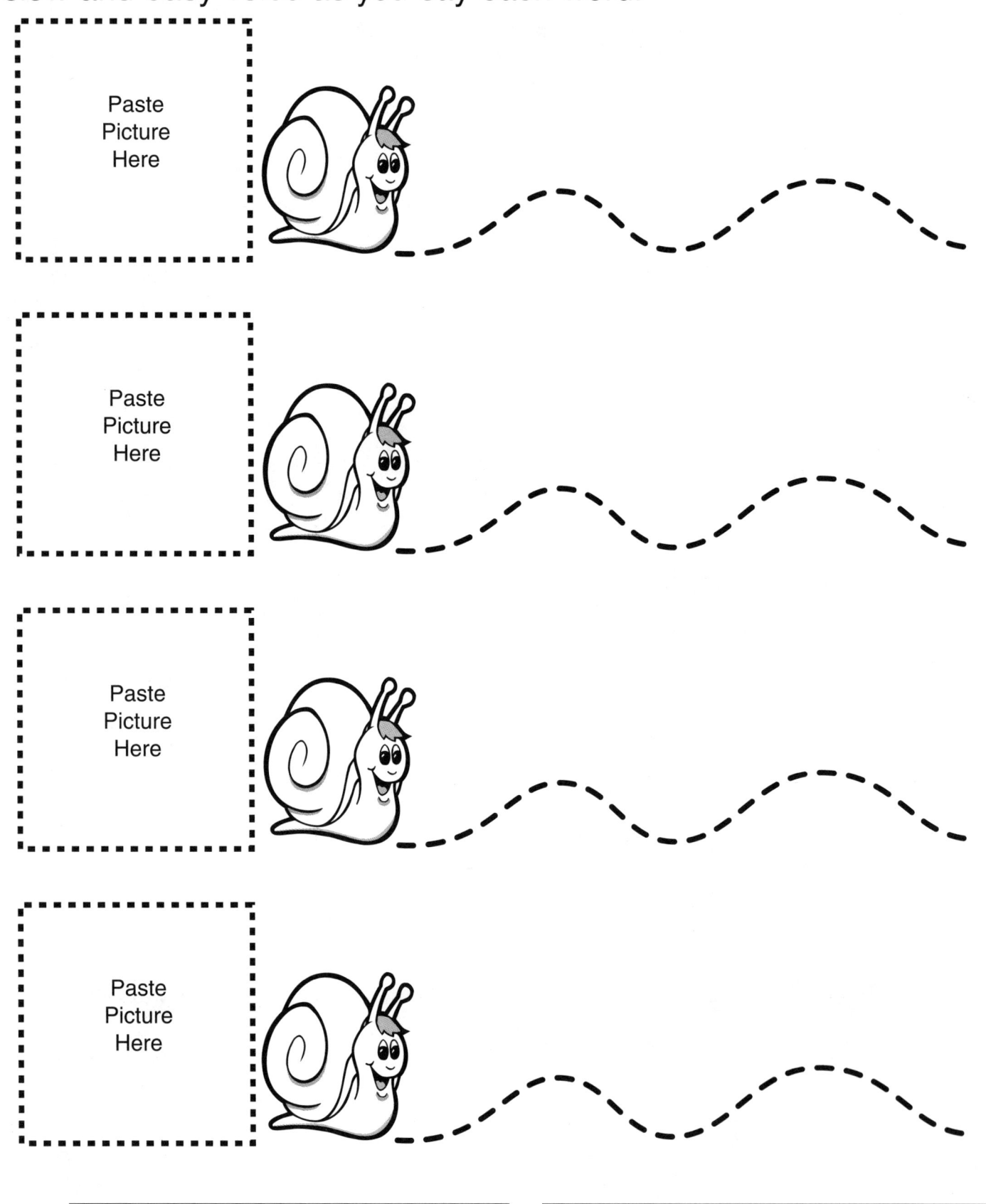

Snooky has fun driving the train! Color, cut and paste your pictures on the train (see pages 76-92). Help Snooky say each word using your slow and easy voice.

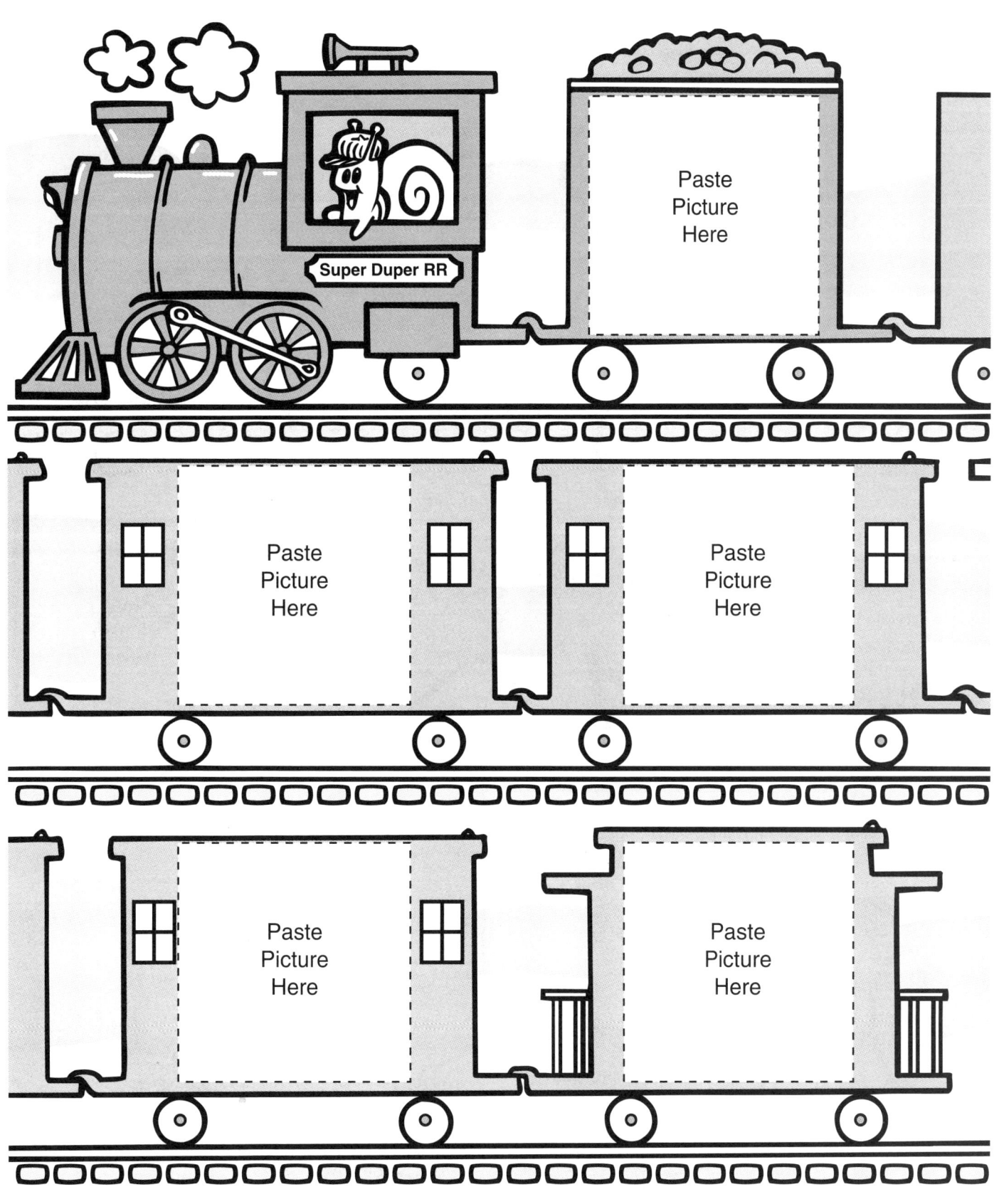

Name   Date   Helper's Signature

Look who Snooky made friends with! Color, cut and paste your pictures on Ollie the Octopus (see pages 76-92). Use your slow and easy voice to help Snooky tell what Ollie is holding.

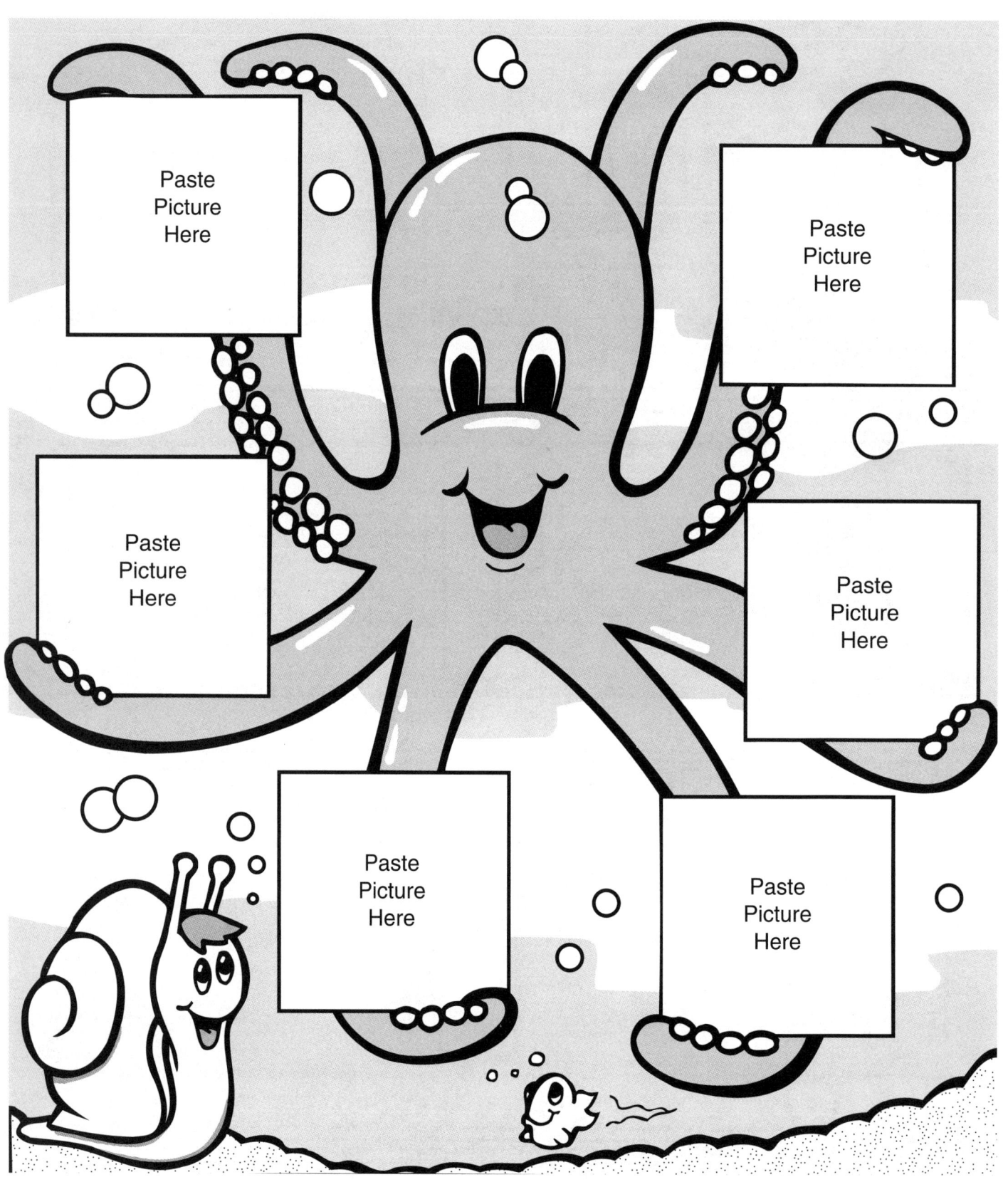

Snooky likes to visit the pond! Color, cut and paste your pictures on the lily pads (see pages 76-92). Use your slow and easy voice to tell Freddy Frog what is on each lily pad.

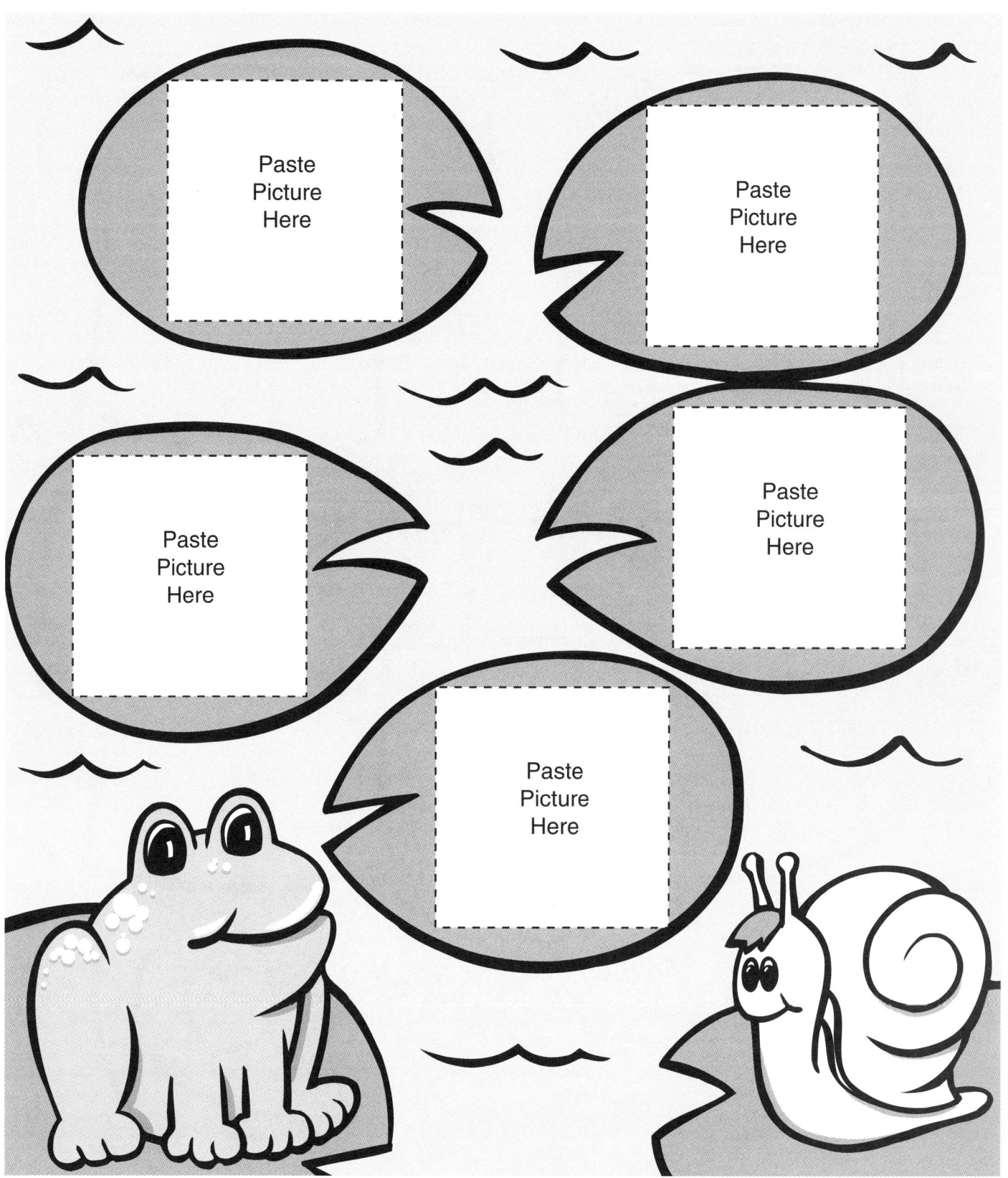

Snooky has been washing clothes. Color, cut and paste your pictures on the T-shirts (see pages 76-92). Tell Snooky, using your slow and easy voice, what the pictures are on the T-shirts.

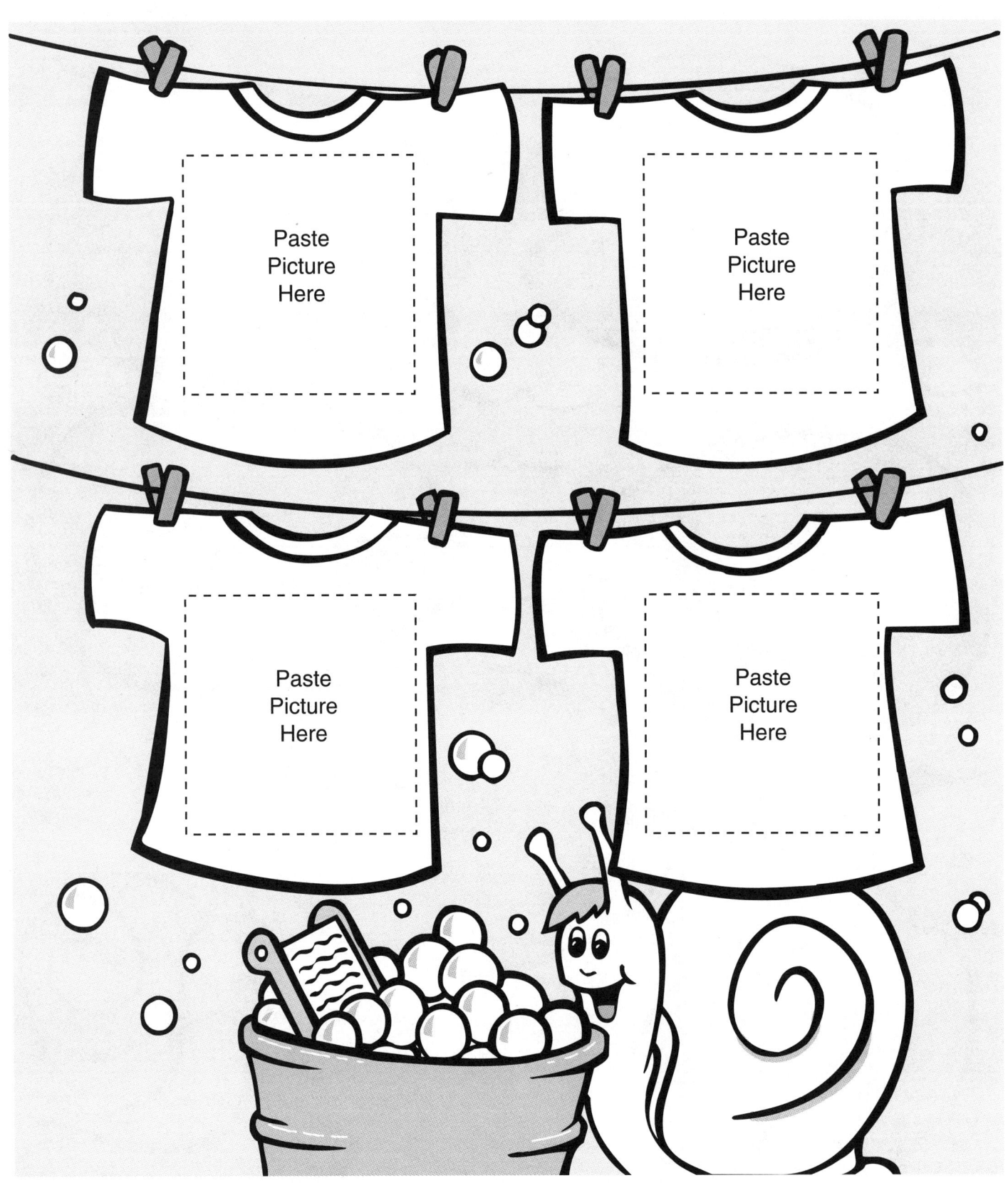

Snooky has tickets to the circus! Color, cut and paste your pictures on the elephants (see pages 76-92). Use your slow and easy voice to tell Snooky what is on each elephant.

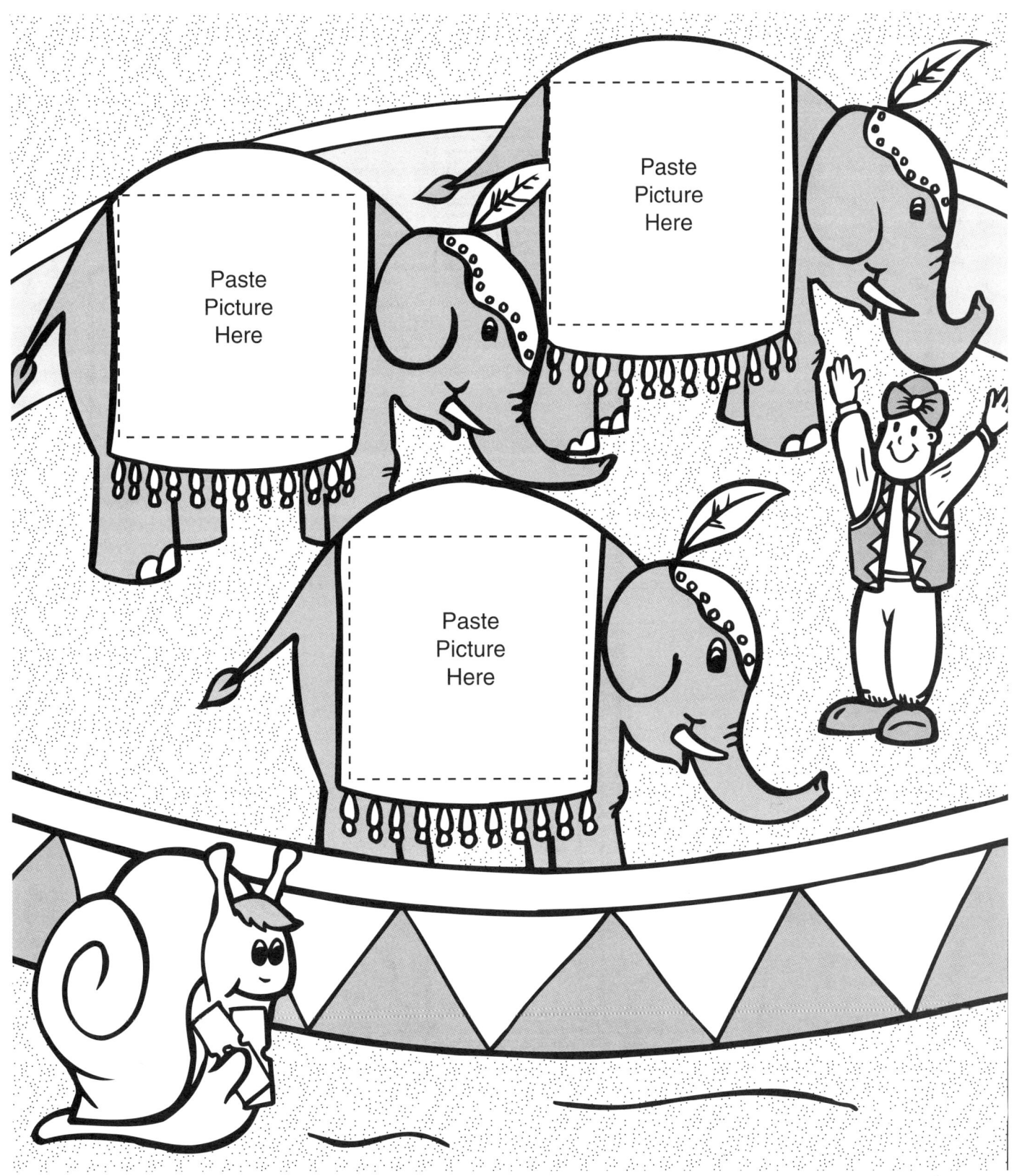

Name _____ Date _____ Helper's Signature _____

15

Snooky enjoys house hunting! Color, cut and paste your pictures on the windows (see pages 76-92). Use your slow and easy voice to tell Snooky what is in each window.

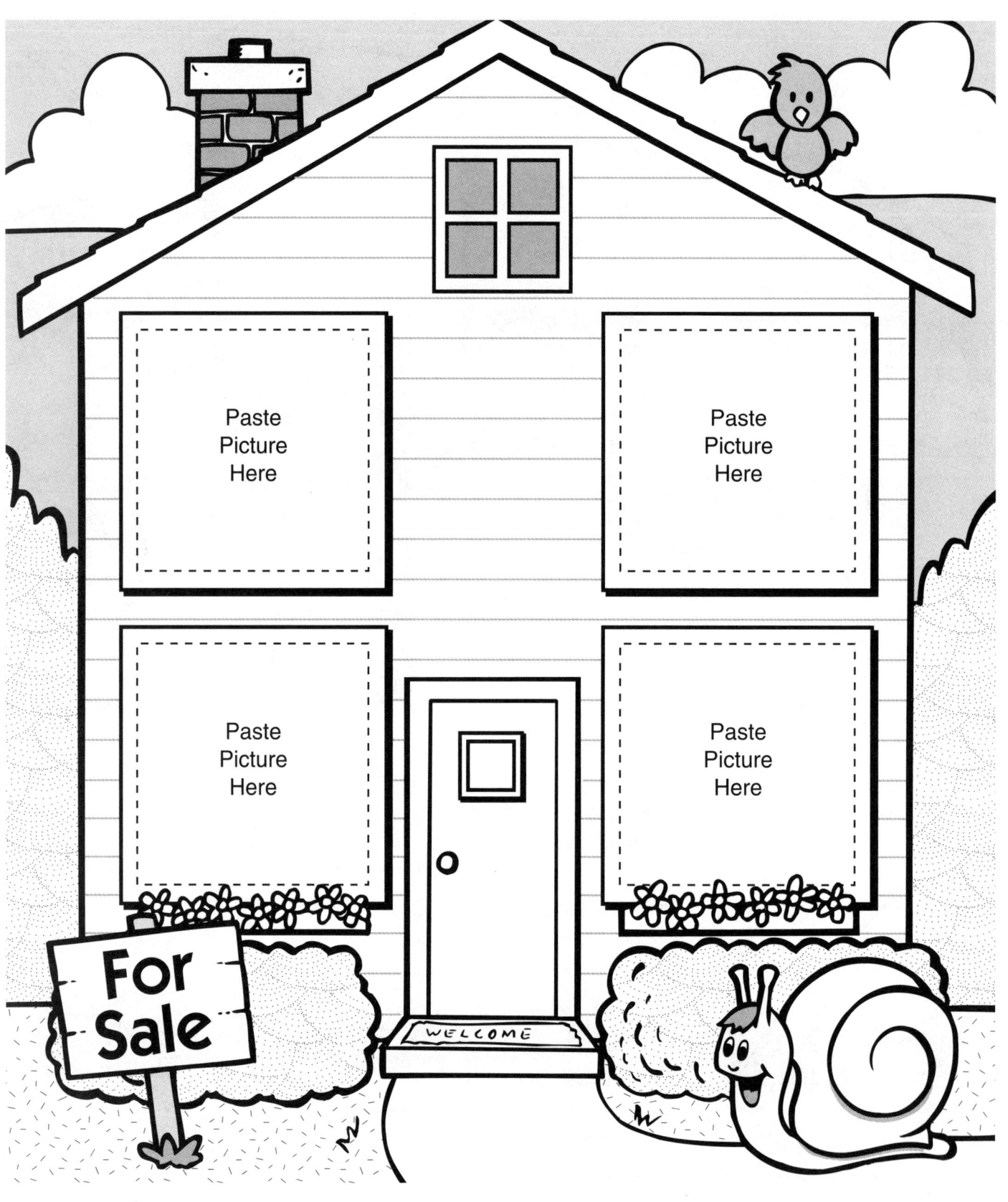

Snooky is blowing speech bubbles! Color, cut and paste your pictures on the bubbles (see pages 76-92). Use your slow and easy voice to tell Snooky what is in each bubble.

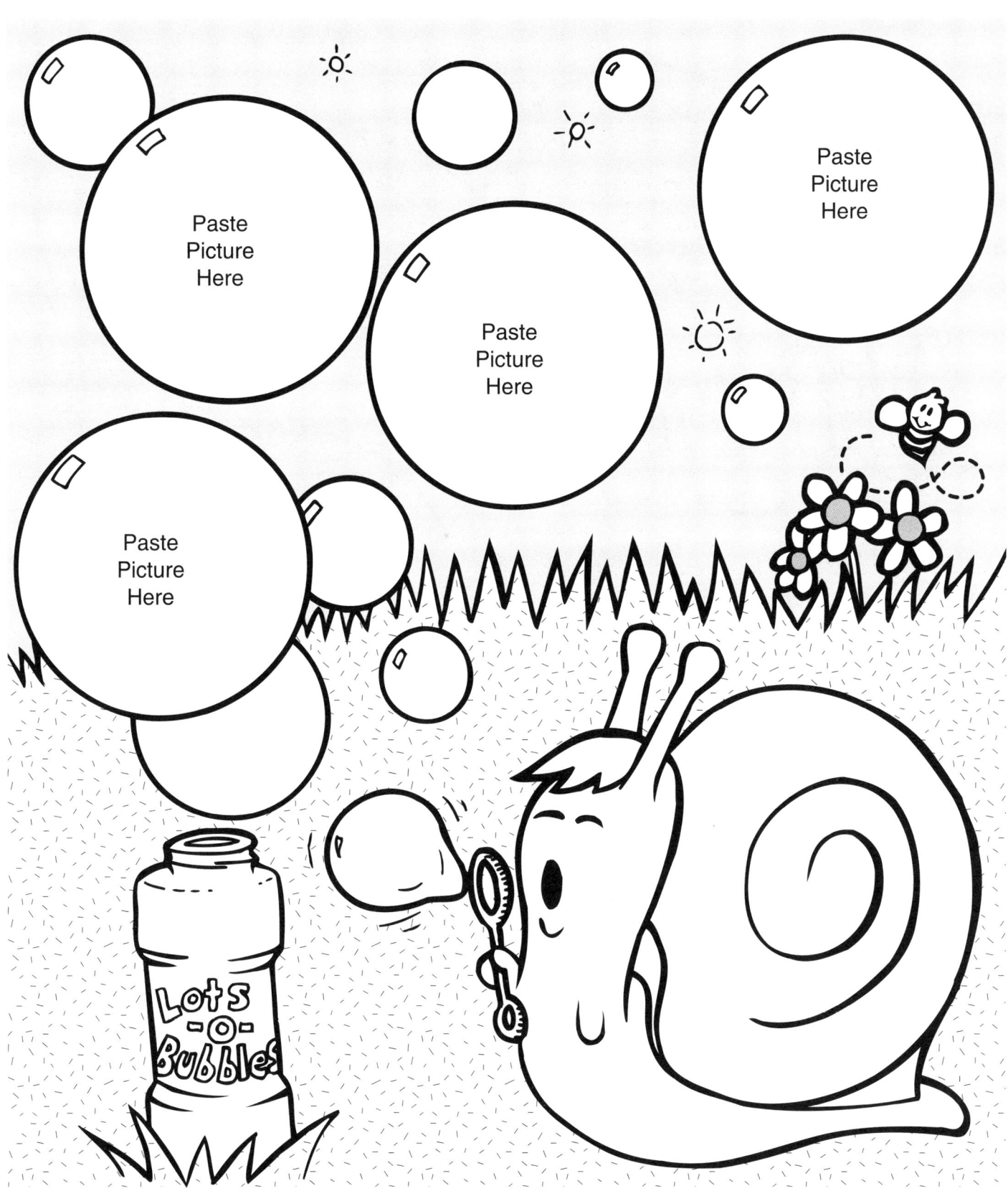

Name _____ Date _____ Helper's Signature _____

Snooky has a friend named Carol Caterpillar. Color, cut and paste your pictures on Carol (see pages 76-92). Use your slow and easy voice to name each picture.

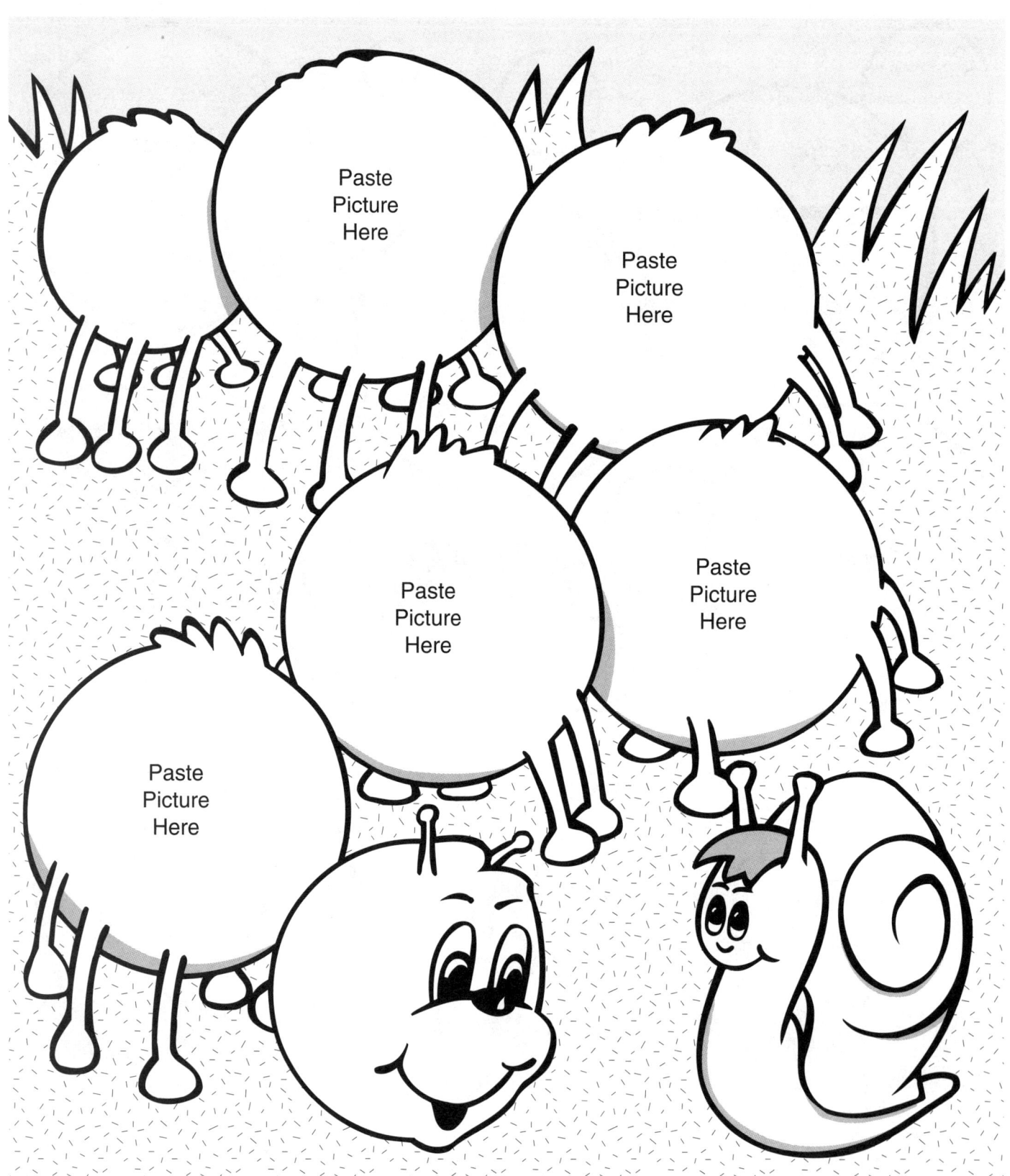

Section 3

Goal: To have child increase utterance length from single words to phrase length when asked a question. A slow and easy voice should be used.

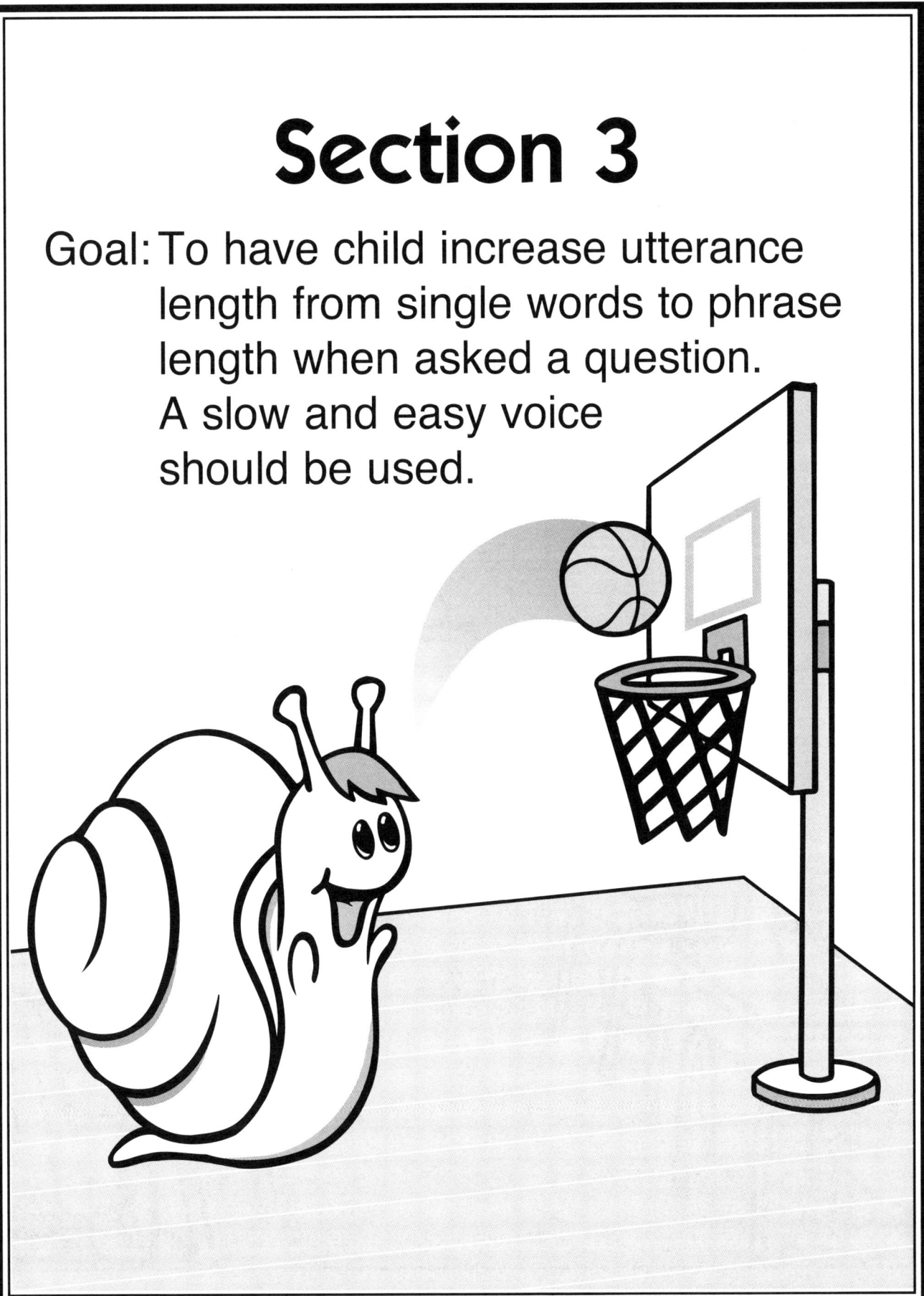

Snooky crawled through your classroom. What did he see? Use your slow and easy voice. Color, cut and paste your pictures on the scene (see page 88).

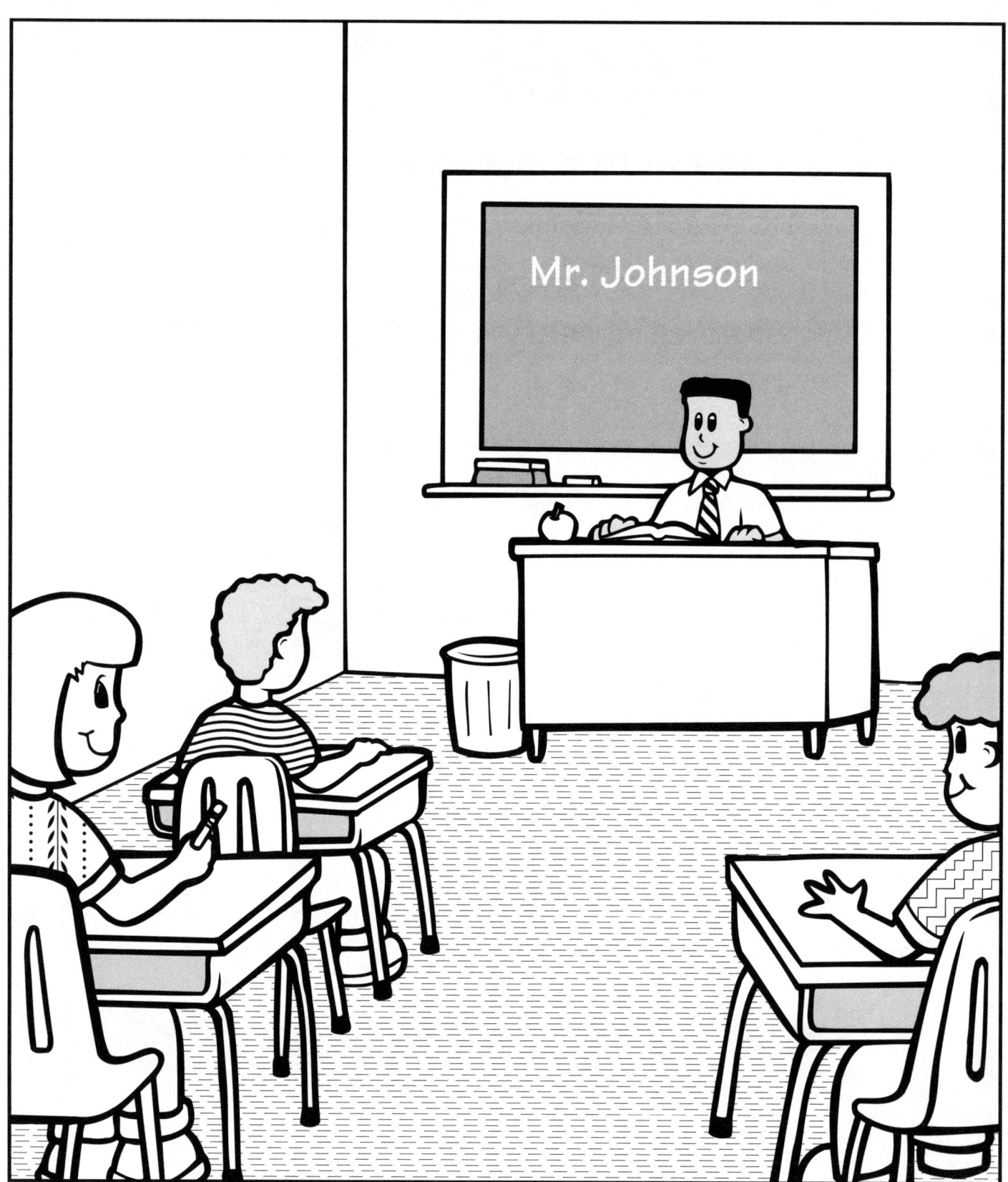

Snooky crawled through the zoo. What did he see? Use your slow and easy voice. Color, cut and paste your pictures on the scene (see page 90).

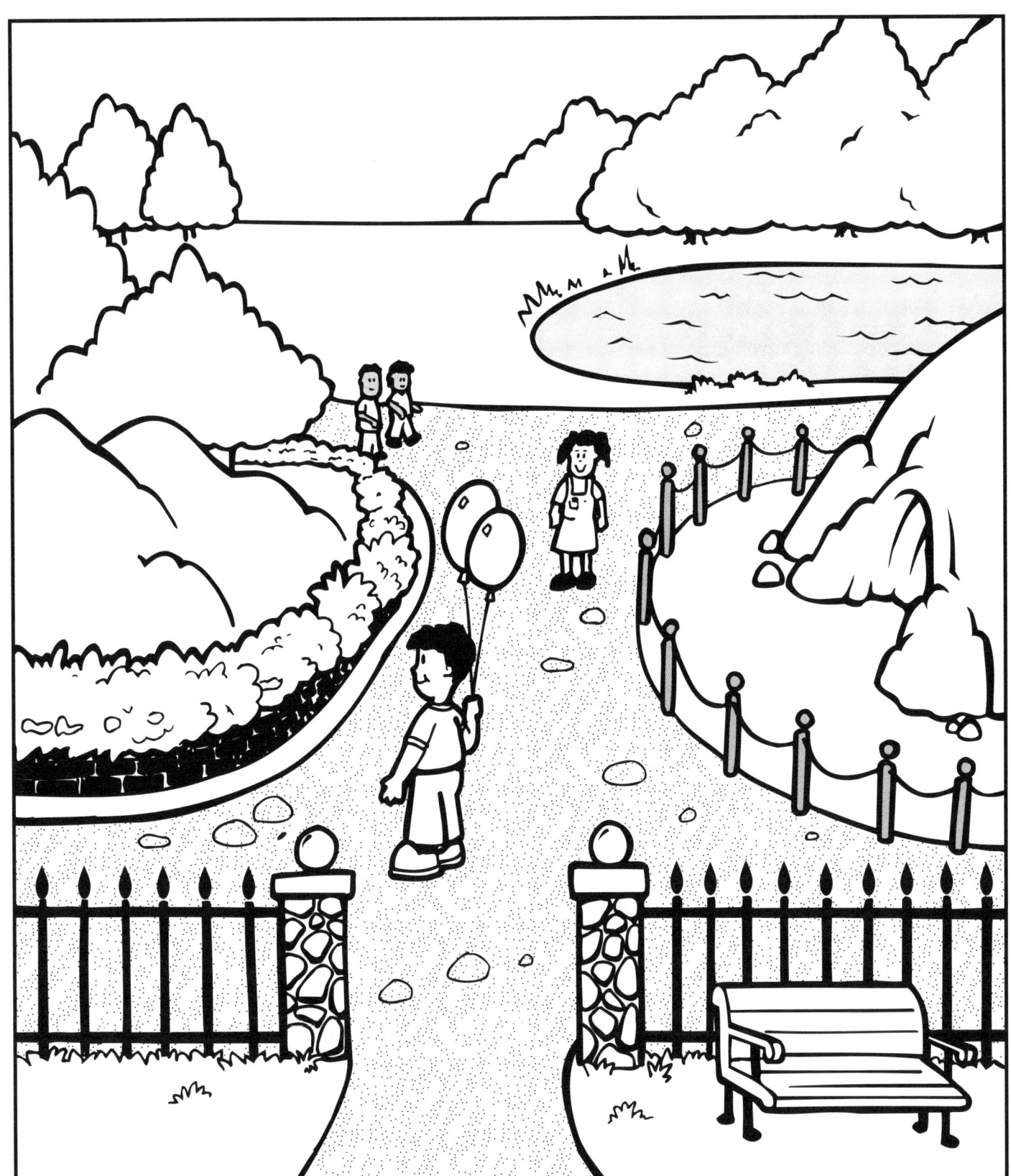

Snooky crawled around the farm. What did he see? Use your slow and easy voice. Color, cut and paste your pictures on the scene (see page 82).

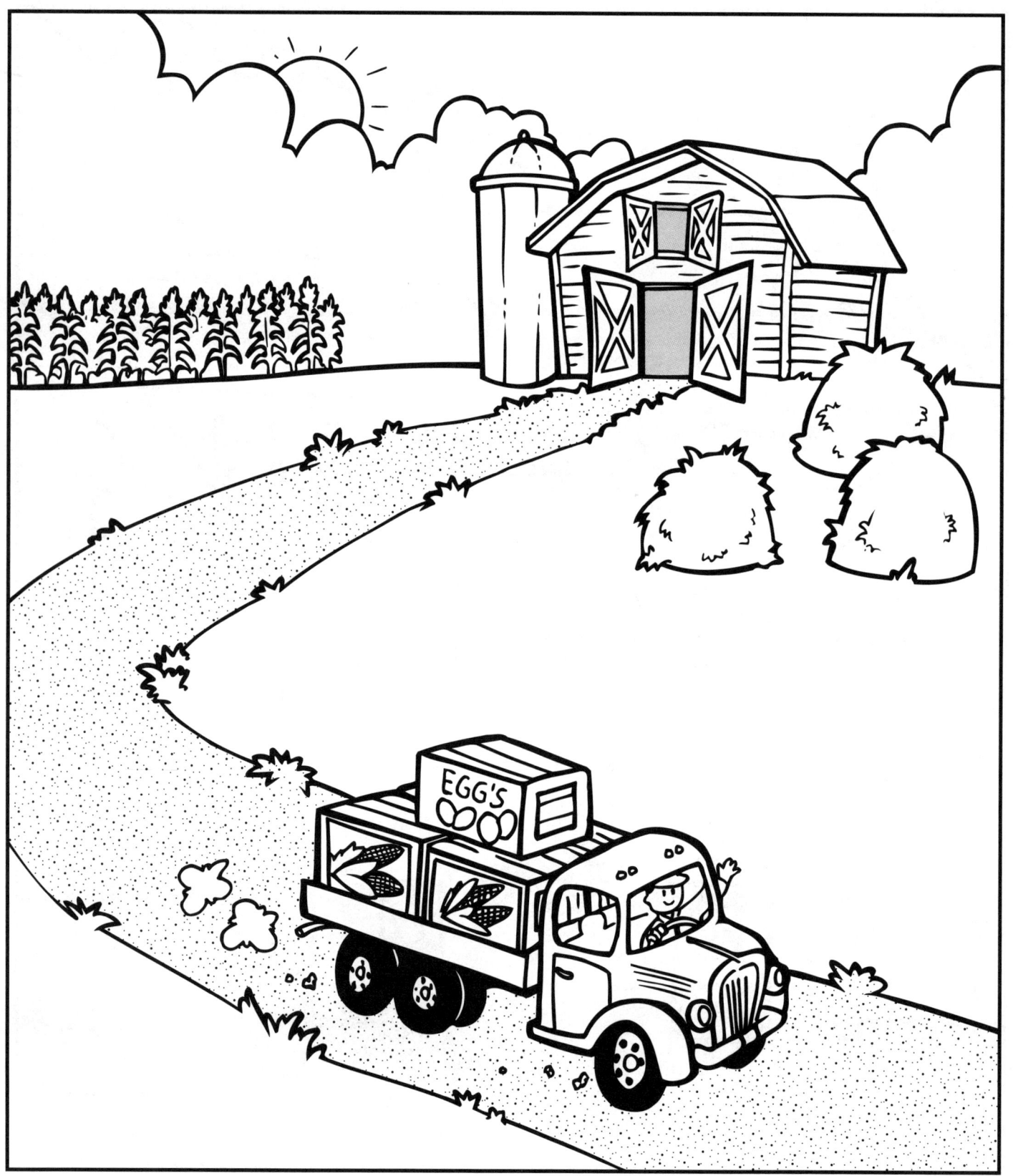

Draw a picture of your family. Name your family members for Snooky using your slow and easy voice. You may also color, cut and paste pictures from page 81.

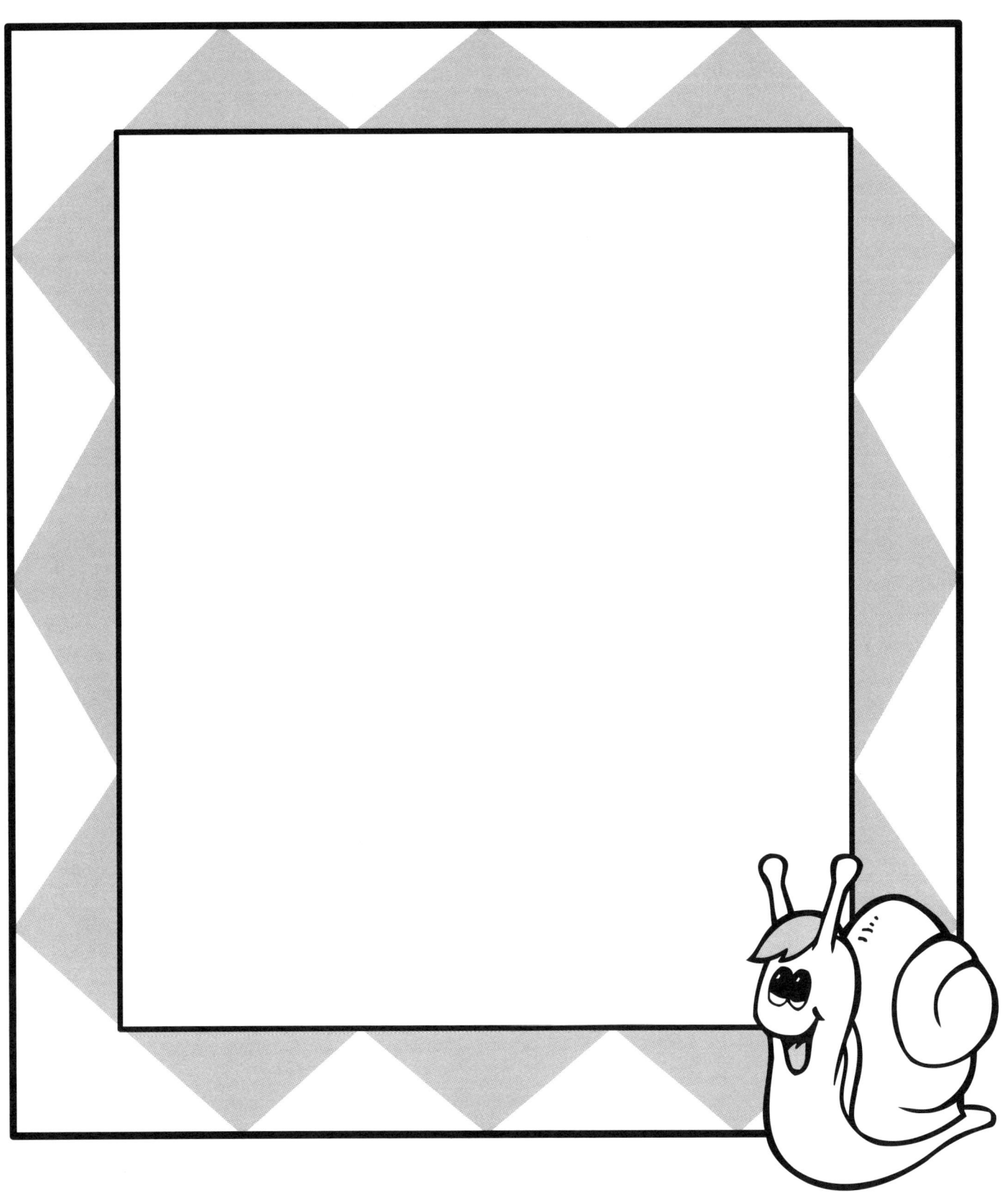

Name _____ Date _____ Helper's Signature _____

Snooky knows all these things are red. What are they? Use your slow and easy voice. Color, cut and paste your pictures on the scene (see page 89).

Name   Date   Helper's Signature

Snooky knows all these things are yellow. What are they? Use your slow and easy voice. Color, cut and paste your pictures on the scene (see page 89).

Name _____ Date _____ Helper's Signature _____

Snooky crawled through your refrigerator. What did he see? Use your slow and easy voice. Color, cut and paste your pictures on the refrigerator (see pages 83-85).

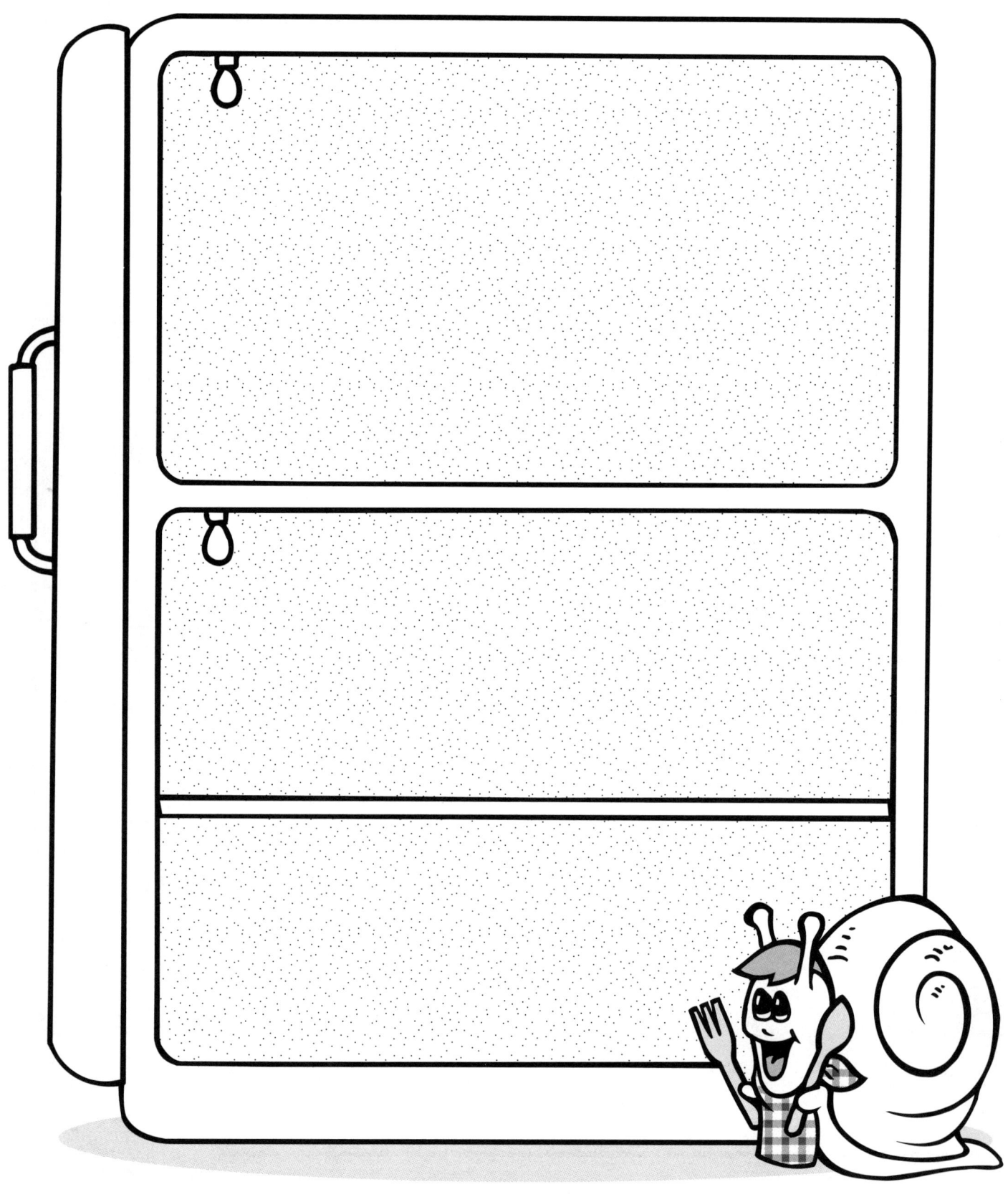

Snooky saw you with your friends. Who did he see? Use your slow and easy voice. Color, cut and paste your pictures on the scene (see page 81).

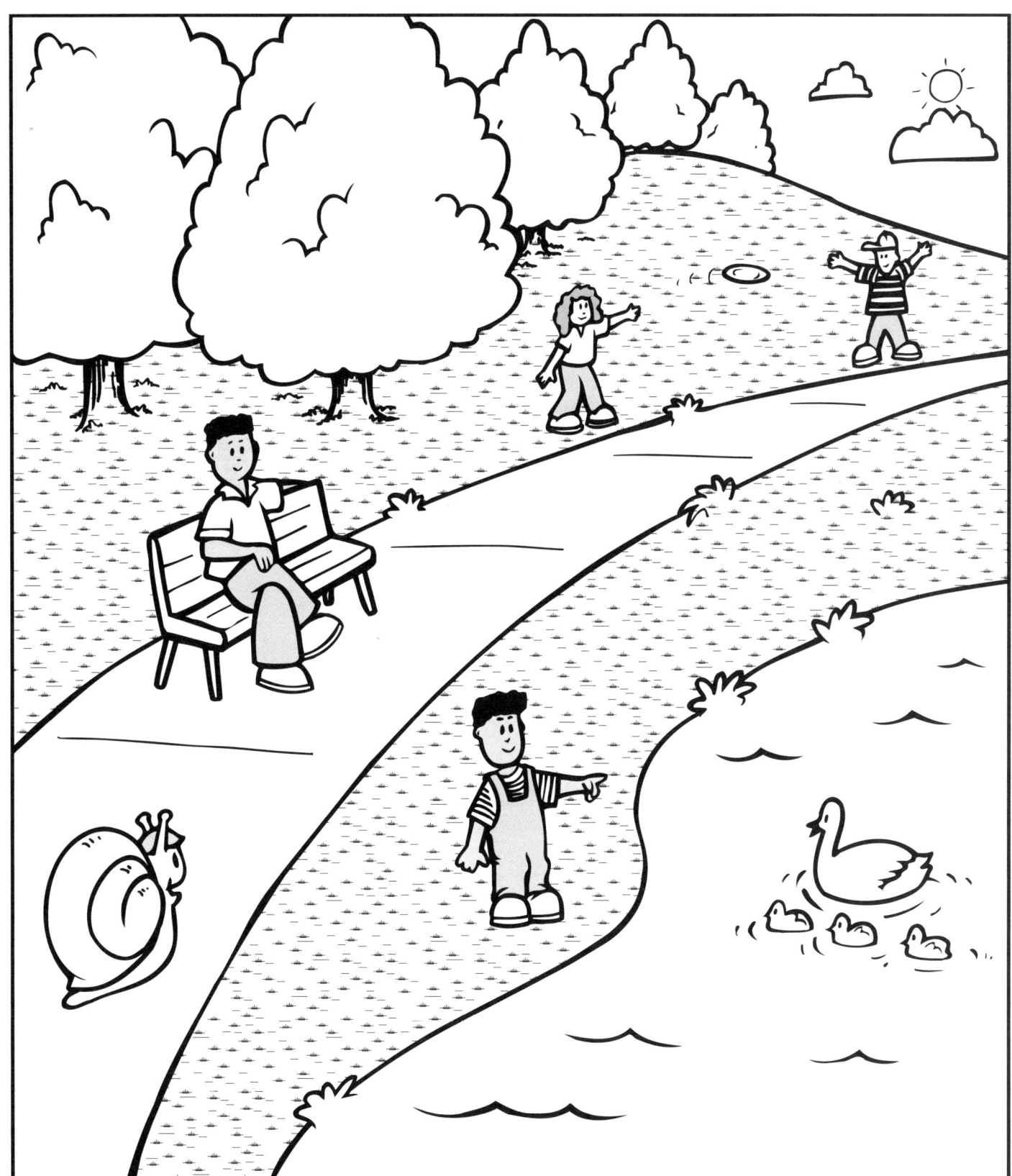

Name Date Helper's Signature

Snooky helped decorate your Christmas tree. What did he put on it? Use your slow and easy voice. Color, cut and paste your pictures on the tree (see page 78).

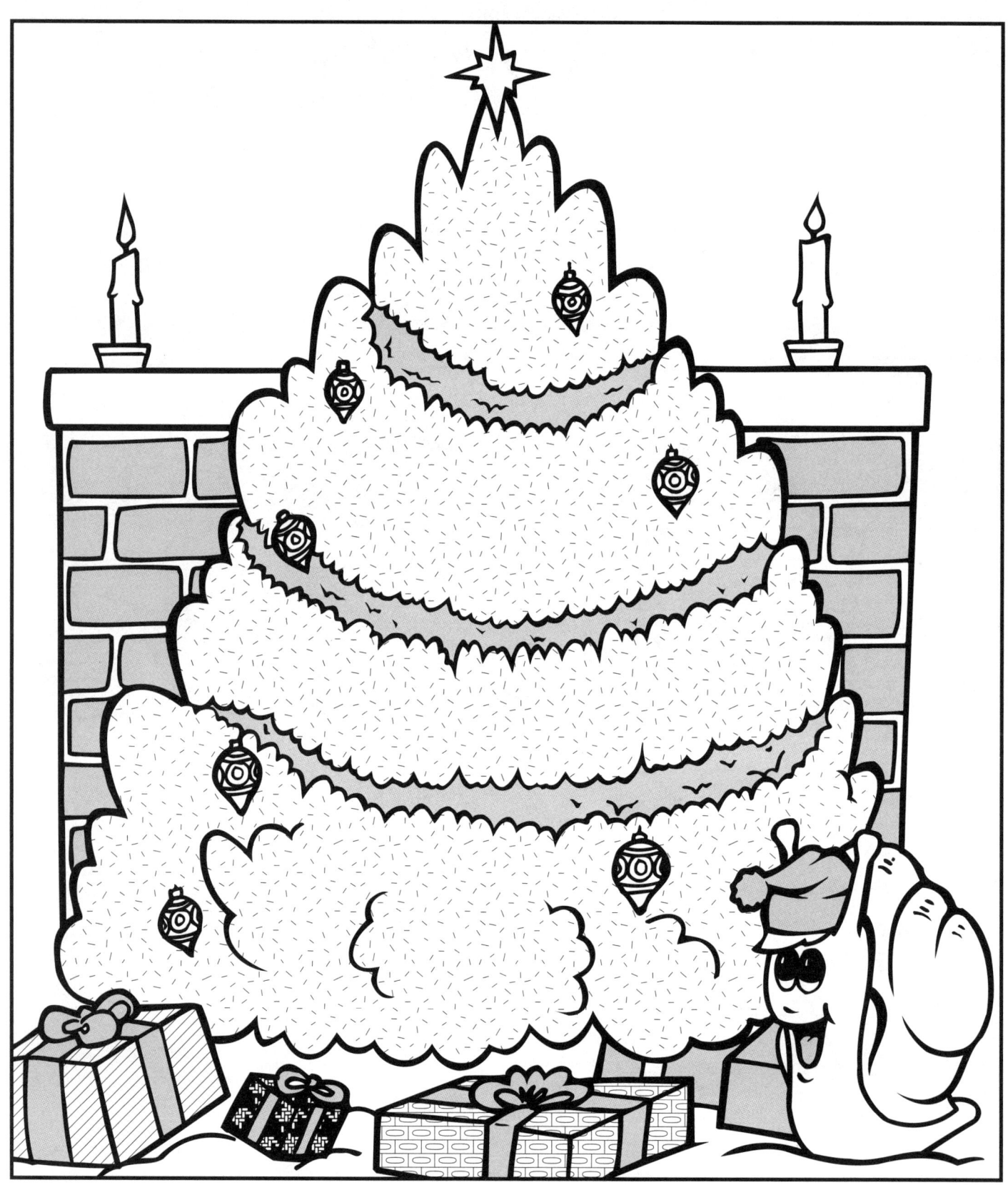

Section 4

Goal: To have child express personal preferences while increasing utterance to sentence level.

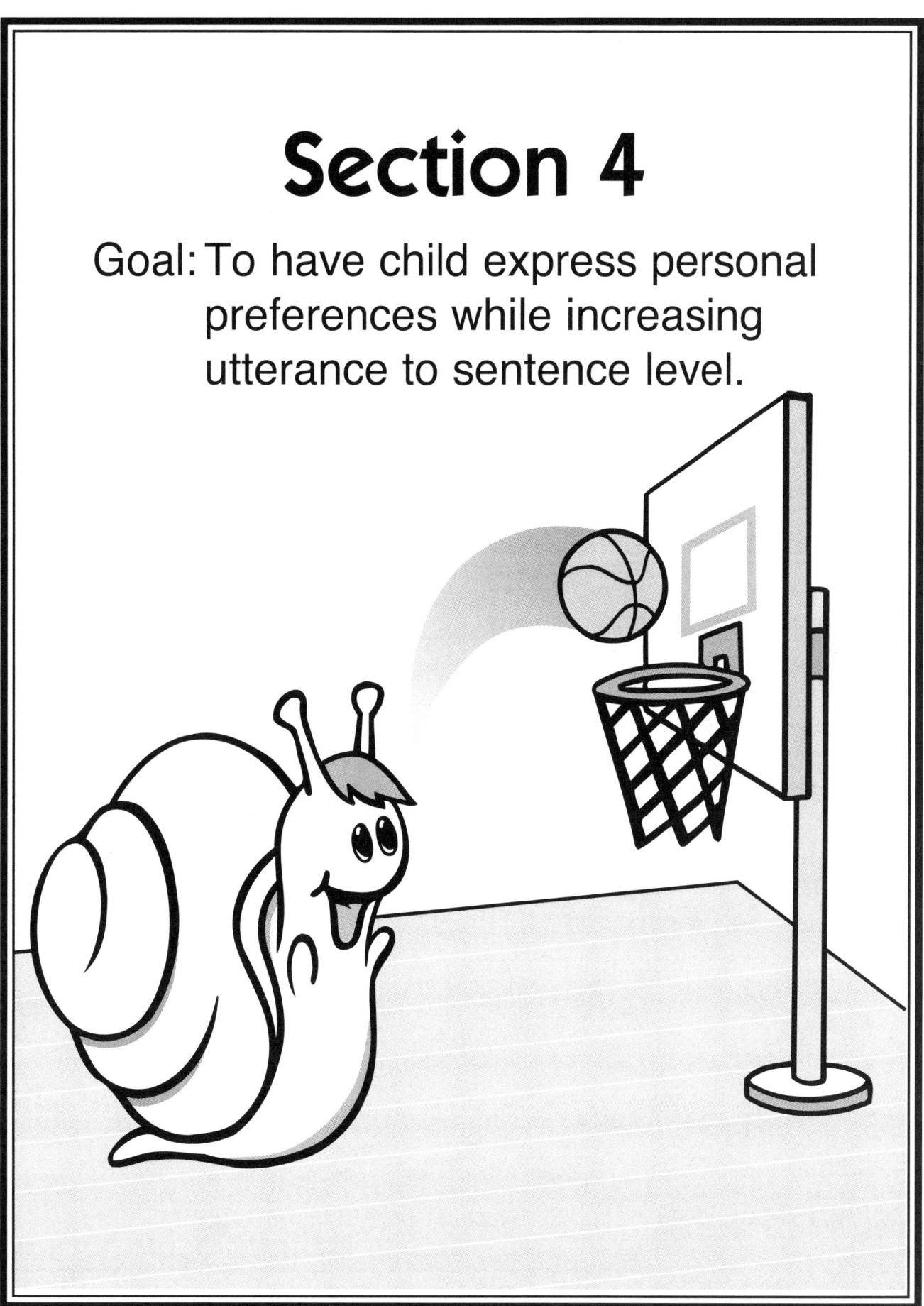

Snooky wants to know what you saw at school. Color, cut and paste your pictures on the scene (see page 88). Use your slow and easy voice when you answer. "I saw a _____."

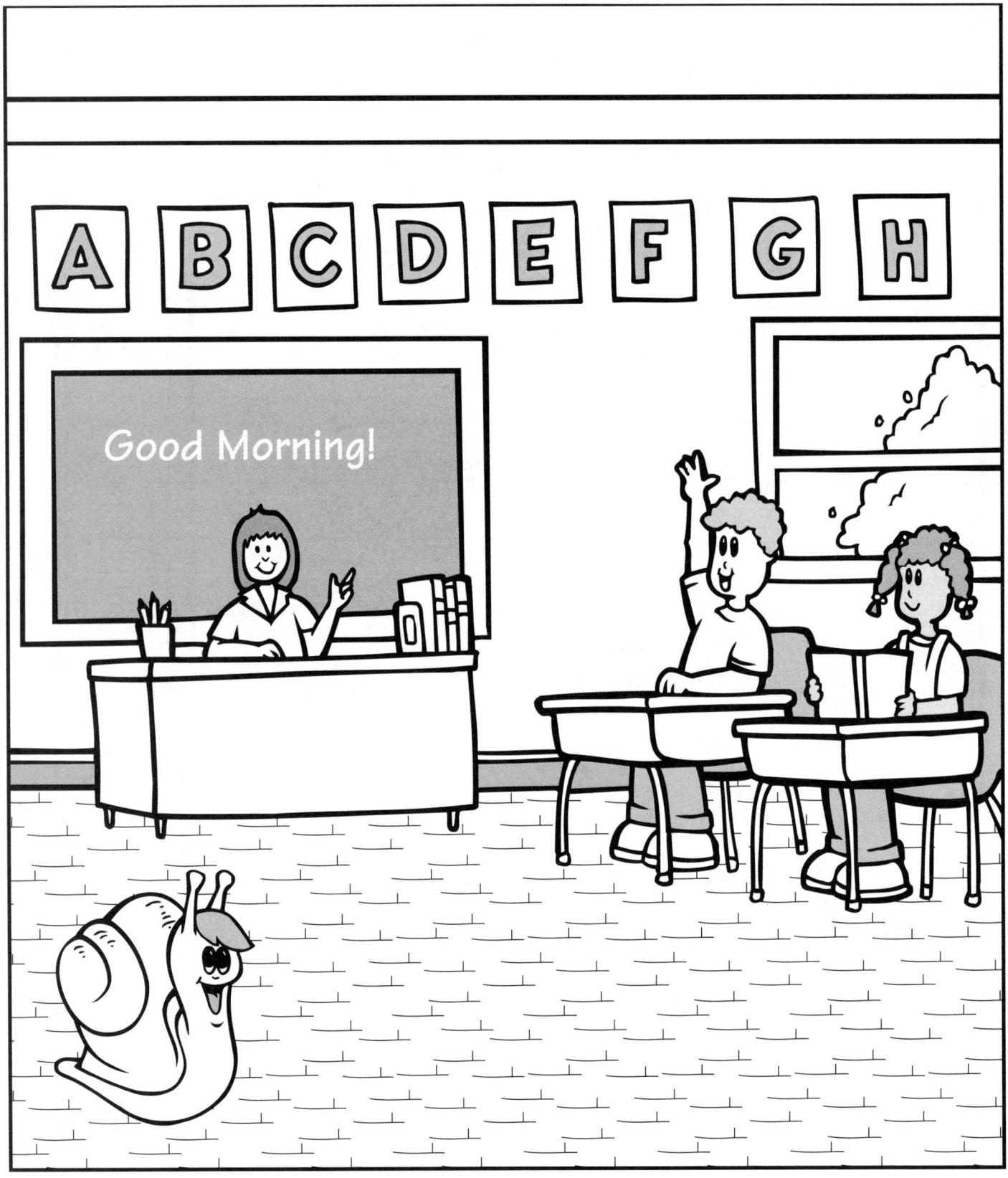

Snooky wants to know what you like to eat. Color, cut and paste your pictures on the scene (see page 83-85). Use your slow and easy voice when you answer. "I like _____."

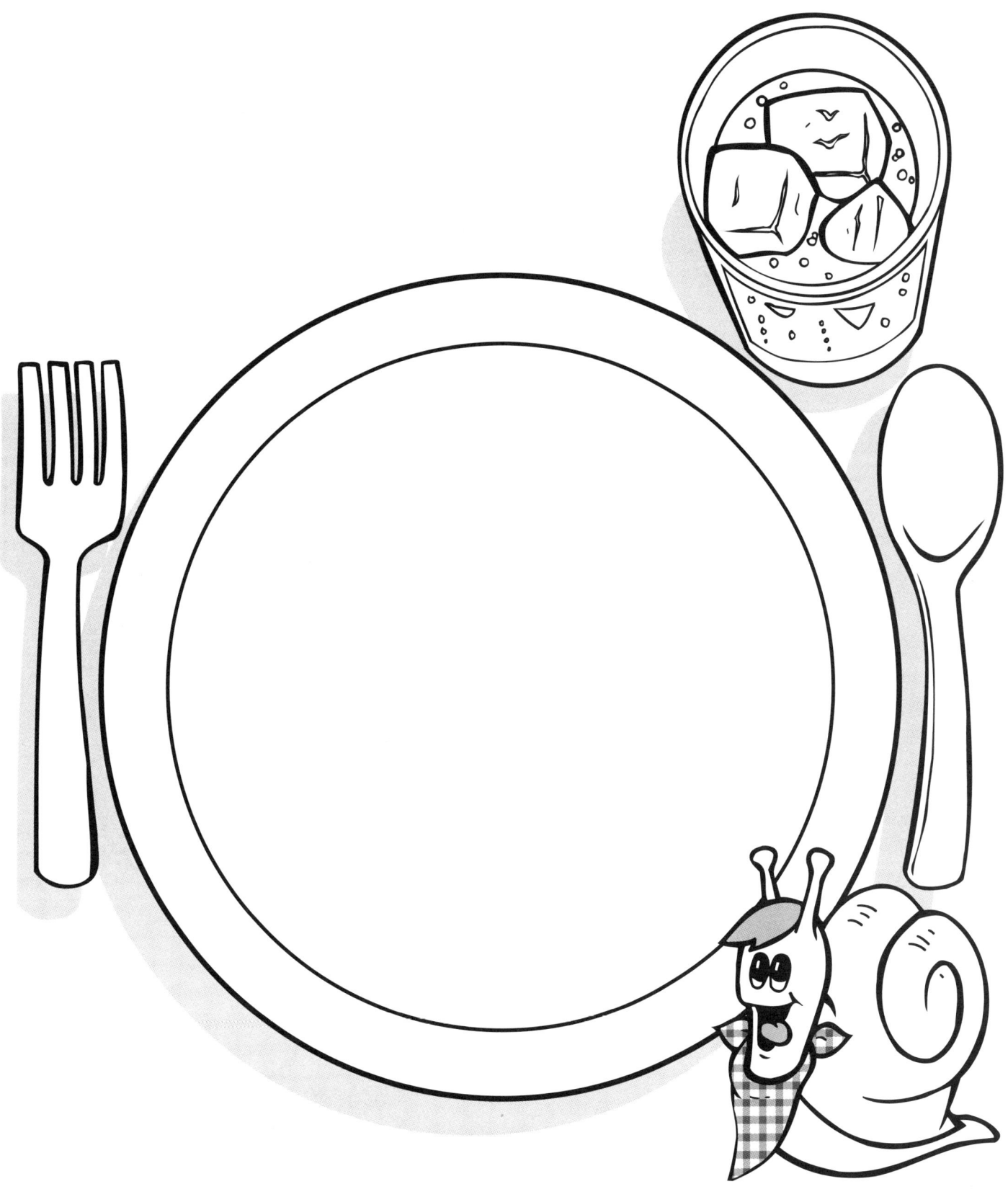

Name   Date   Helper's Signature

Snooky wants to know what you can do at the playground. Color, cut and paste your pictures on the scene (see page 87). Use your slow and easy voice when you answer. "I can _____."

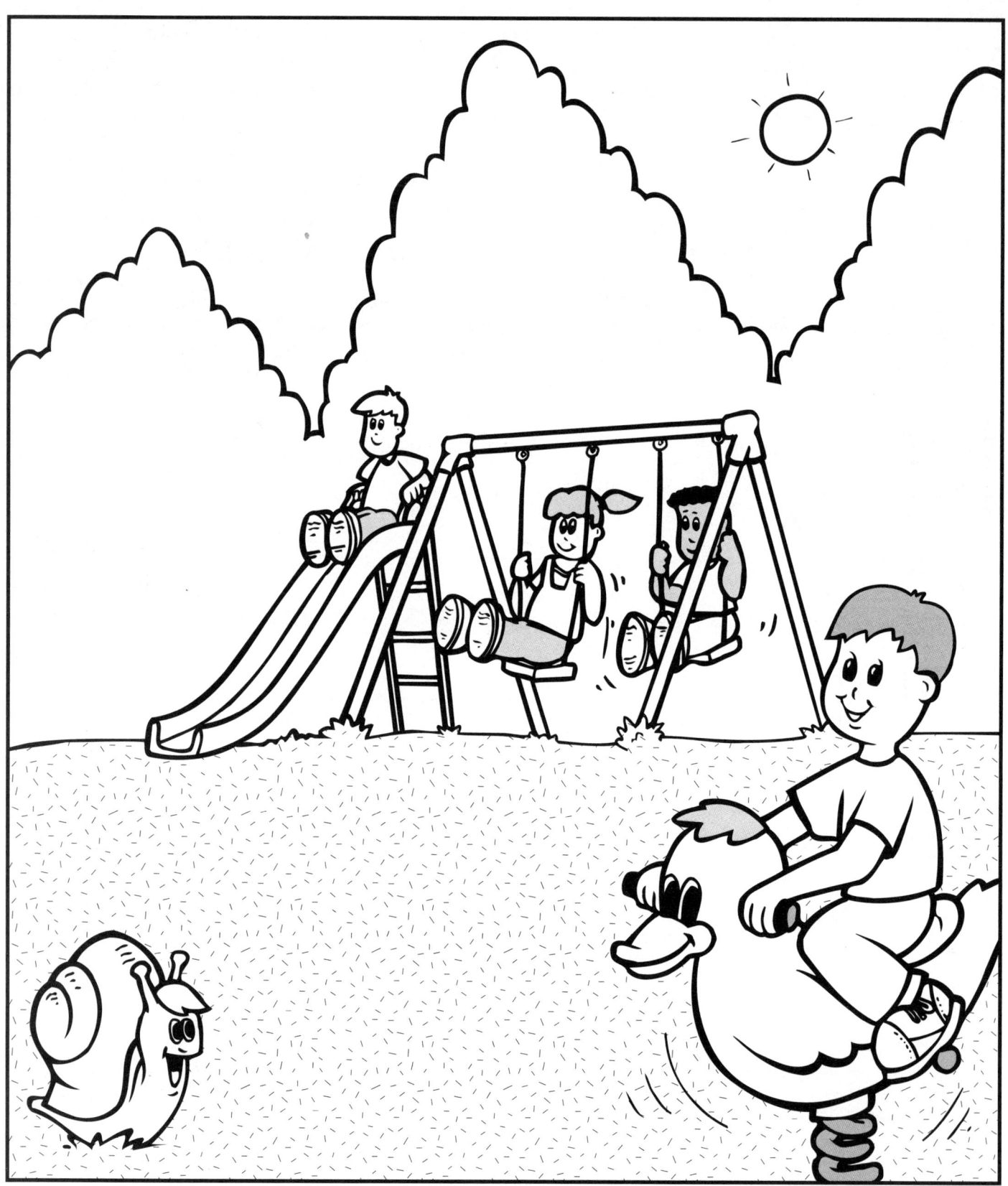

Snooky wants to know what you bought when you went shopping. Color, cut and paste your pictures on the scene (see pages 83-86). Use your slow and easy voice when you answer. "I bought _____."

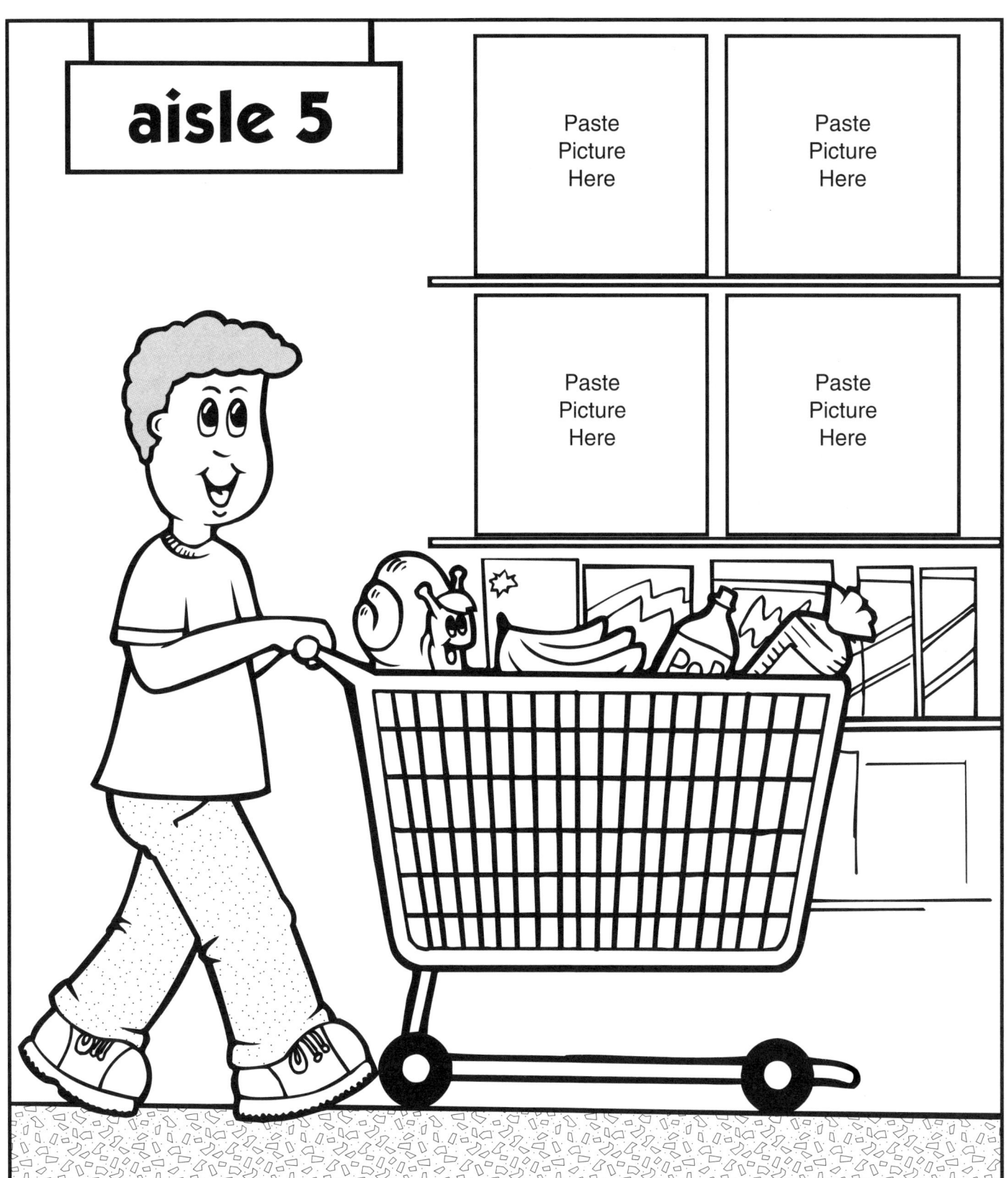

Snooky wants to know what you have in your toy box. Color, cut and paste your pictures on the toy box (see page 87). Use your slow and easy voice when you answer. "I have _____."

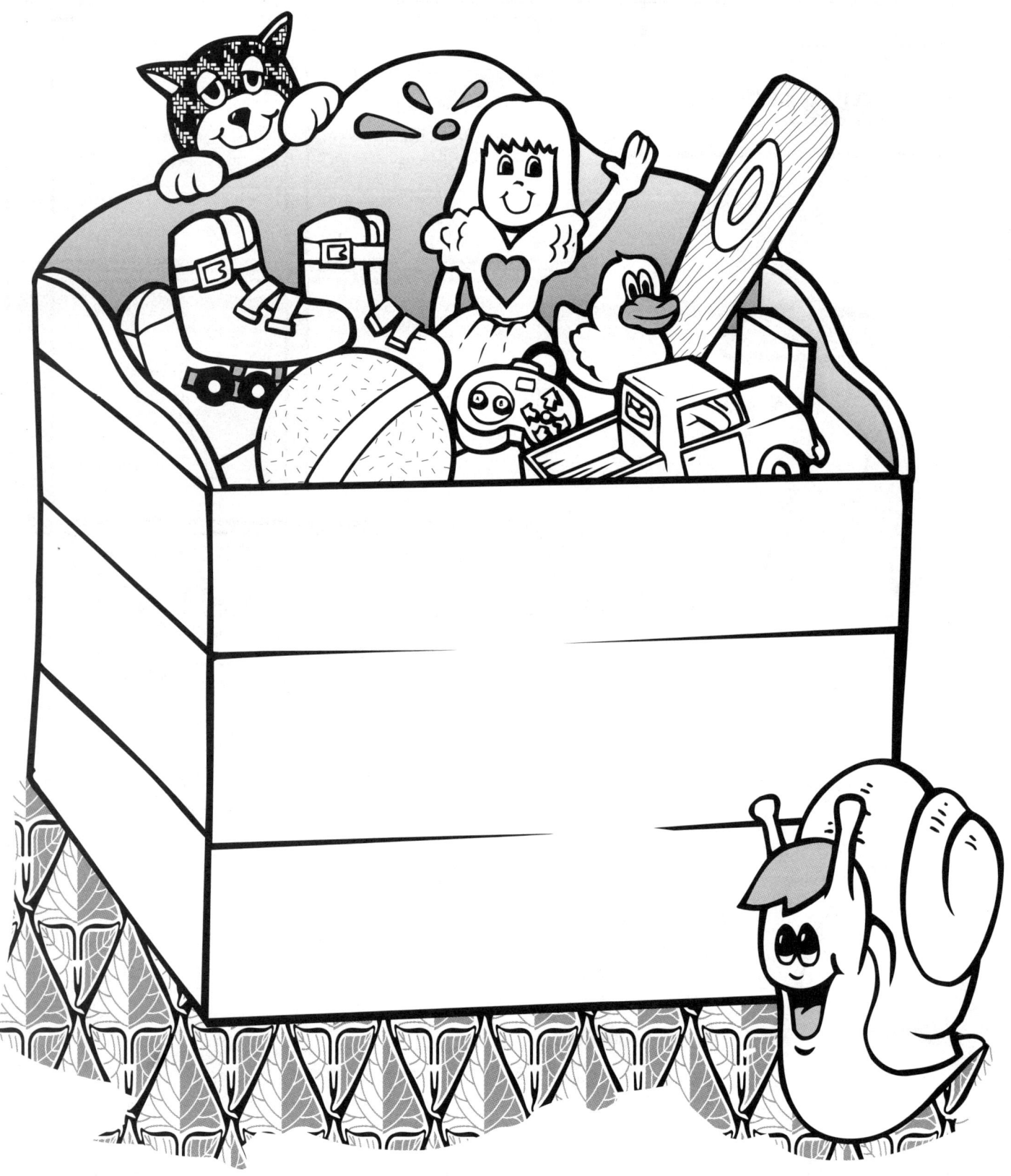

Snooky wants to know what you want for your birthday. Color, cut and paste your pictures on the scene (see page 87). Use your slow and easy voice when you answer. "I want _____."

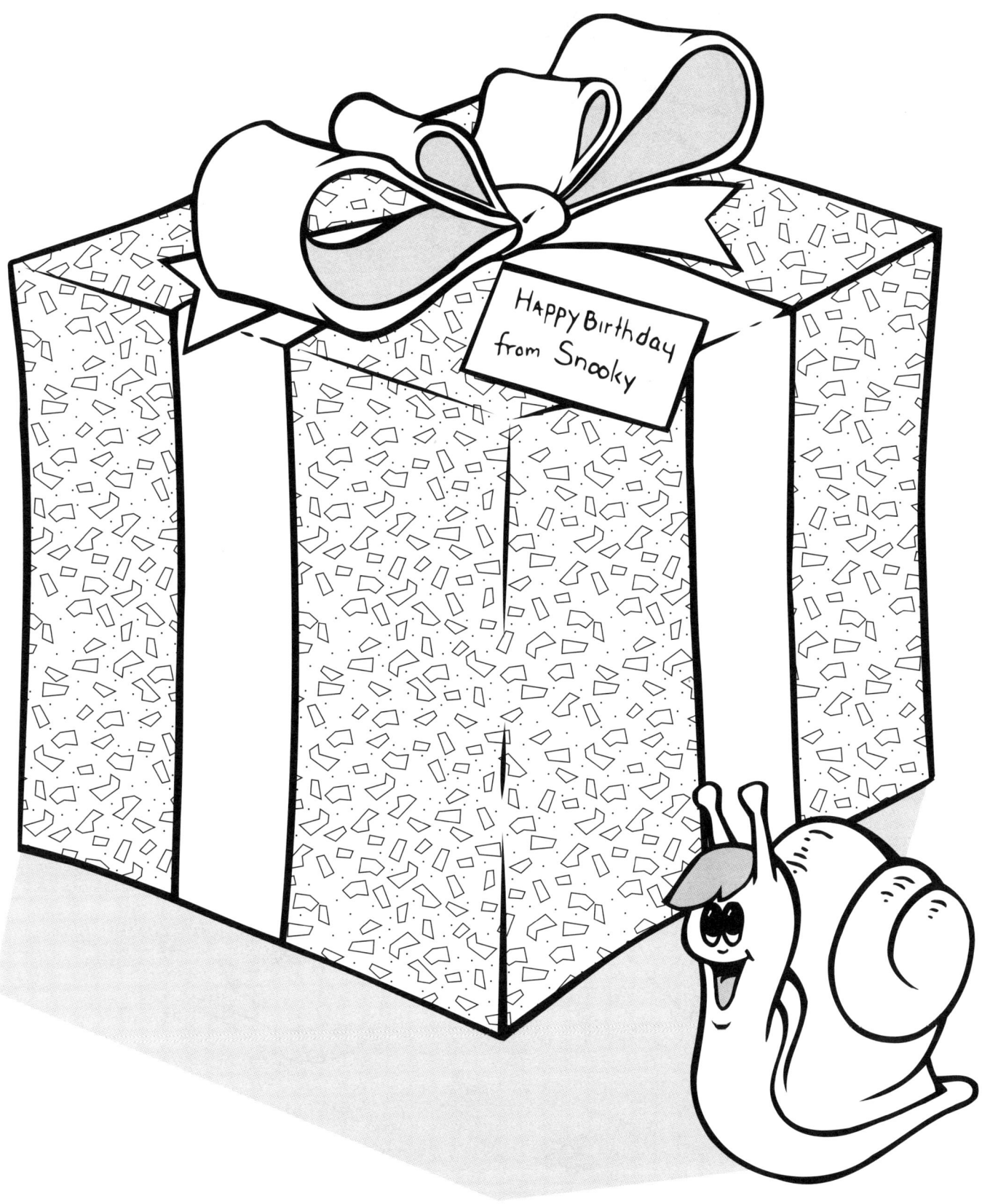

_____   _____   _____
Name   Date   Helper's Signature

Snooky wants to know what you wear when it is hot outside. Color, cut and paste your pictures on the scene (see page 80). Use your slow and easy voice when you answer. "I wear _____."

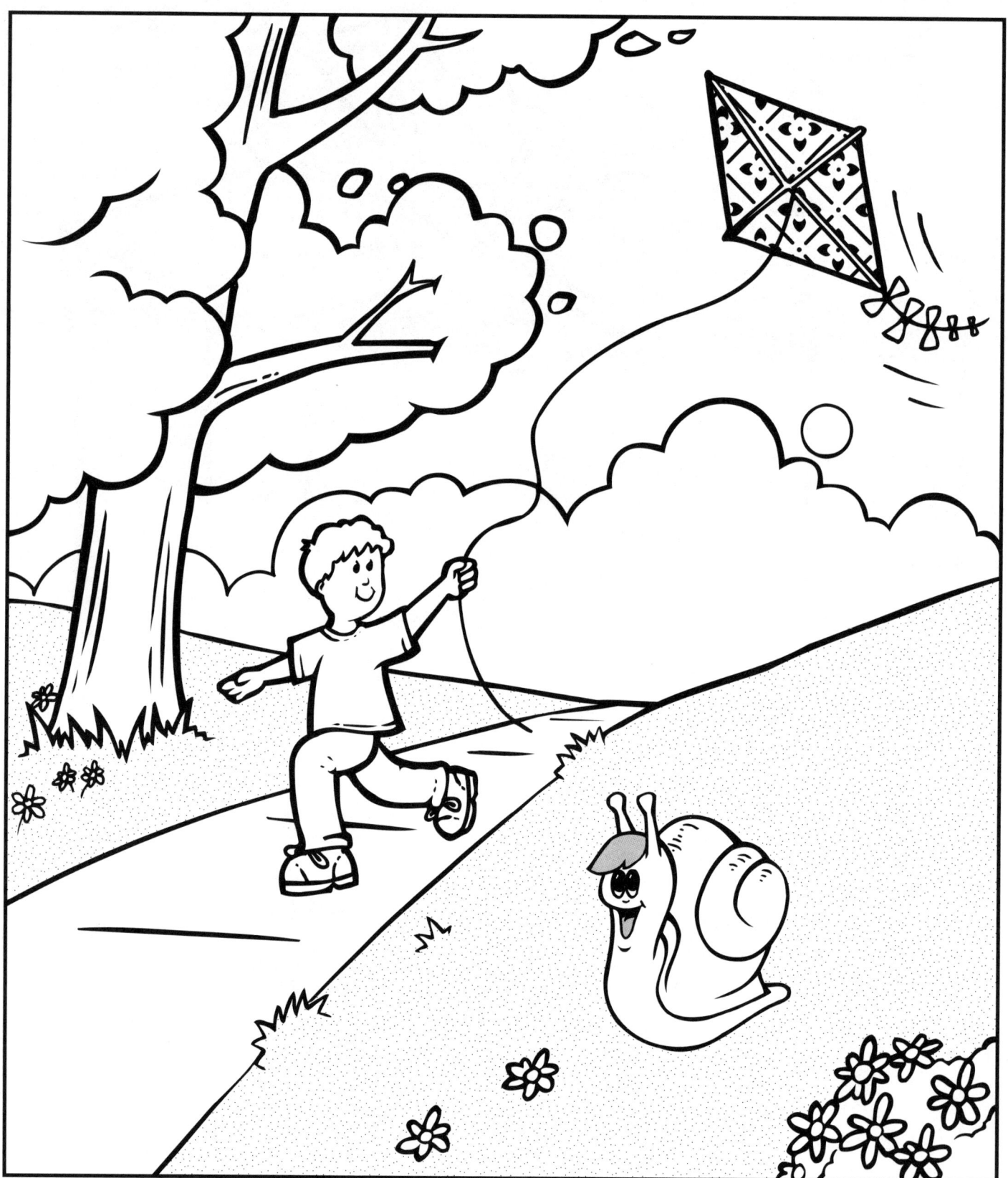

Snooky wants to know what you wear when it is cold outside. Color, cut and paste your pictures on the scene (see page 80). Use your slow and easy voice when you answer. "I wear _____."

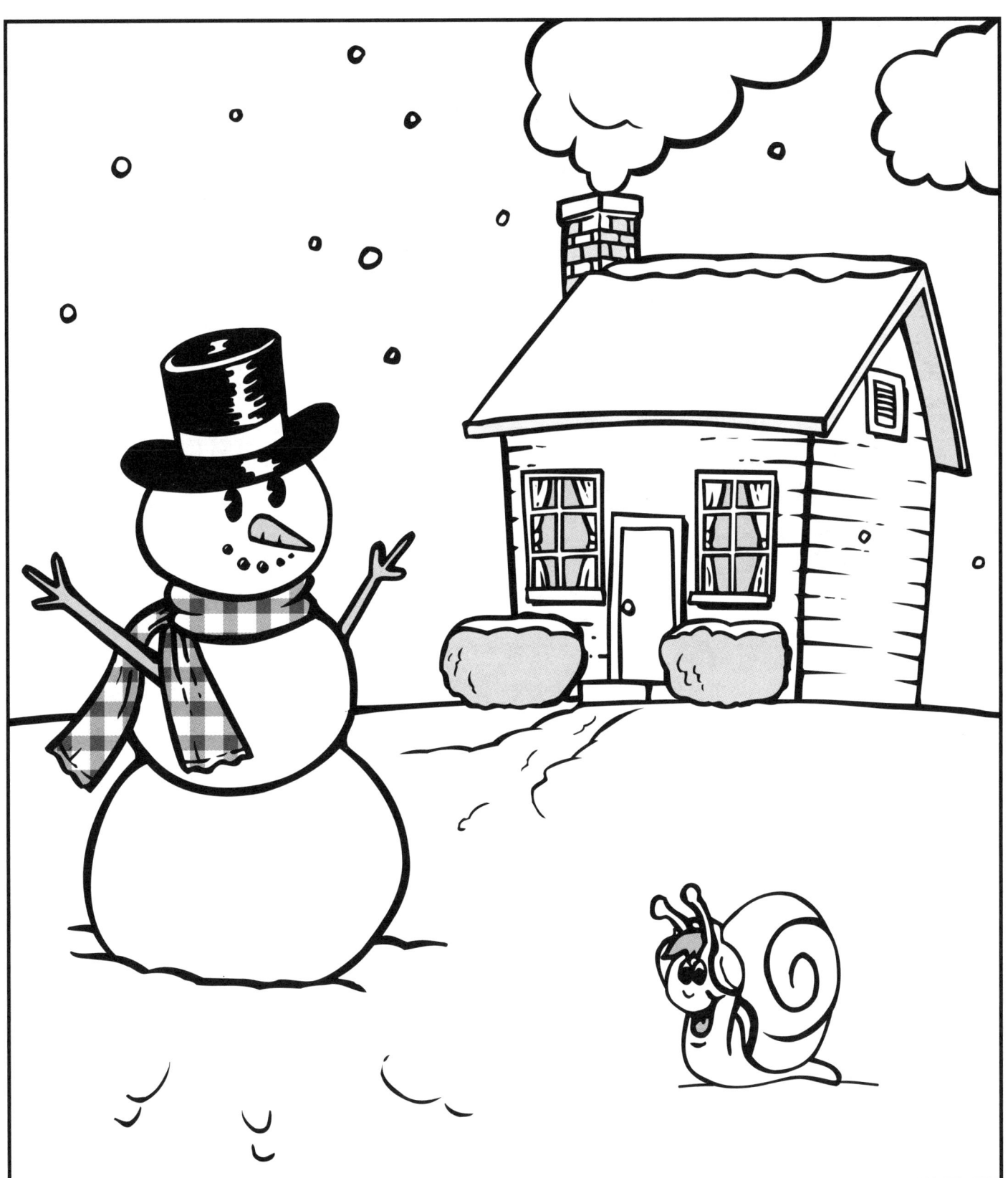

Snooky wants to know what you saw at the zoo. Color, cut and paste your pictures on the scene (see page 90). Use your slow and easy voice when you answer. "I saw _____."

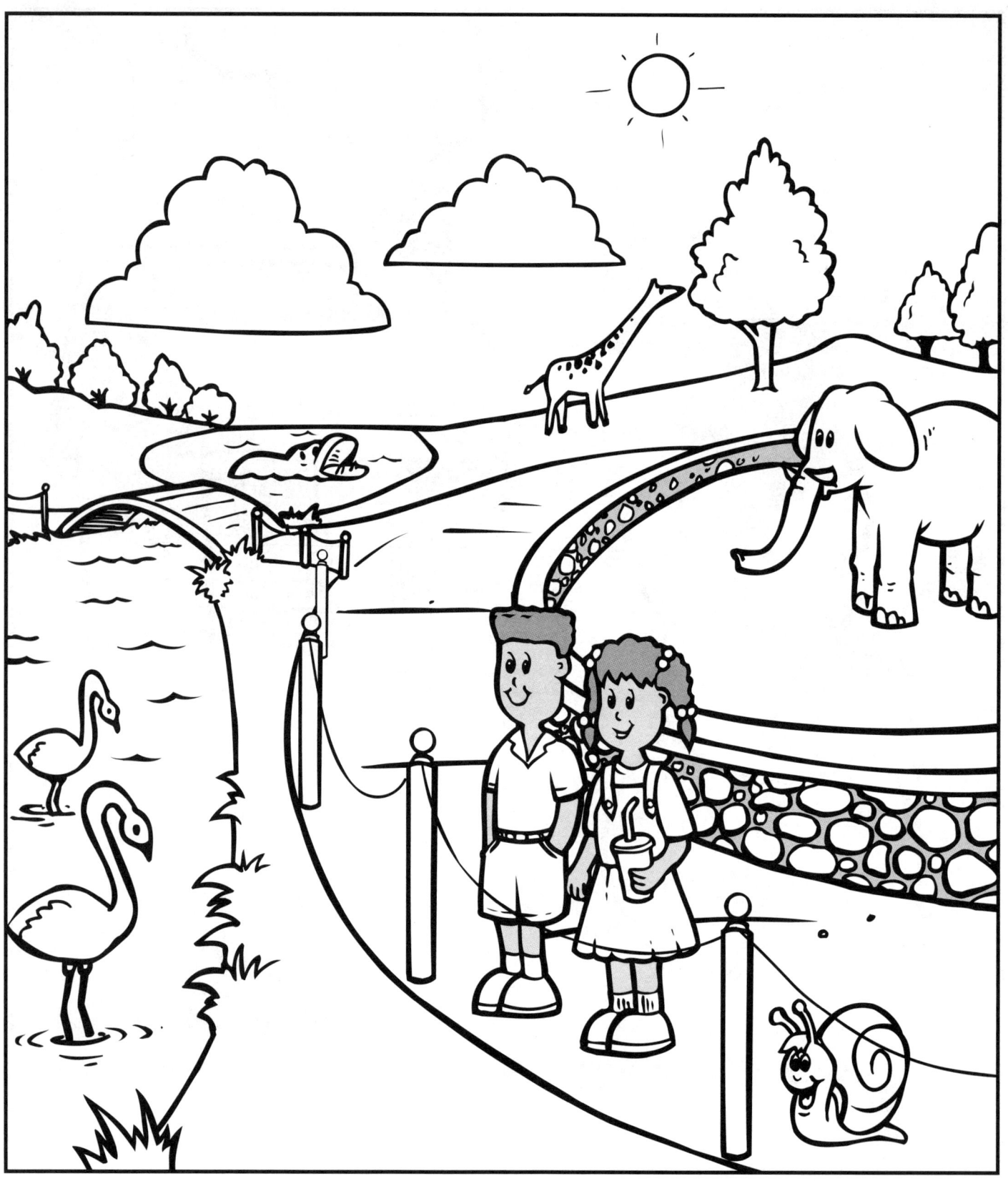

Section 5

Goal: To have child increase length of sentence utterances by answering Snooky Snail's questions. A slow and easy voice should be used.

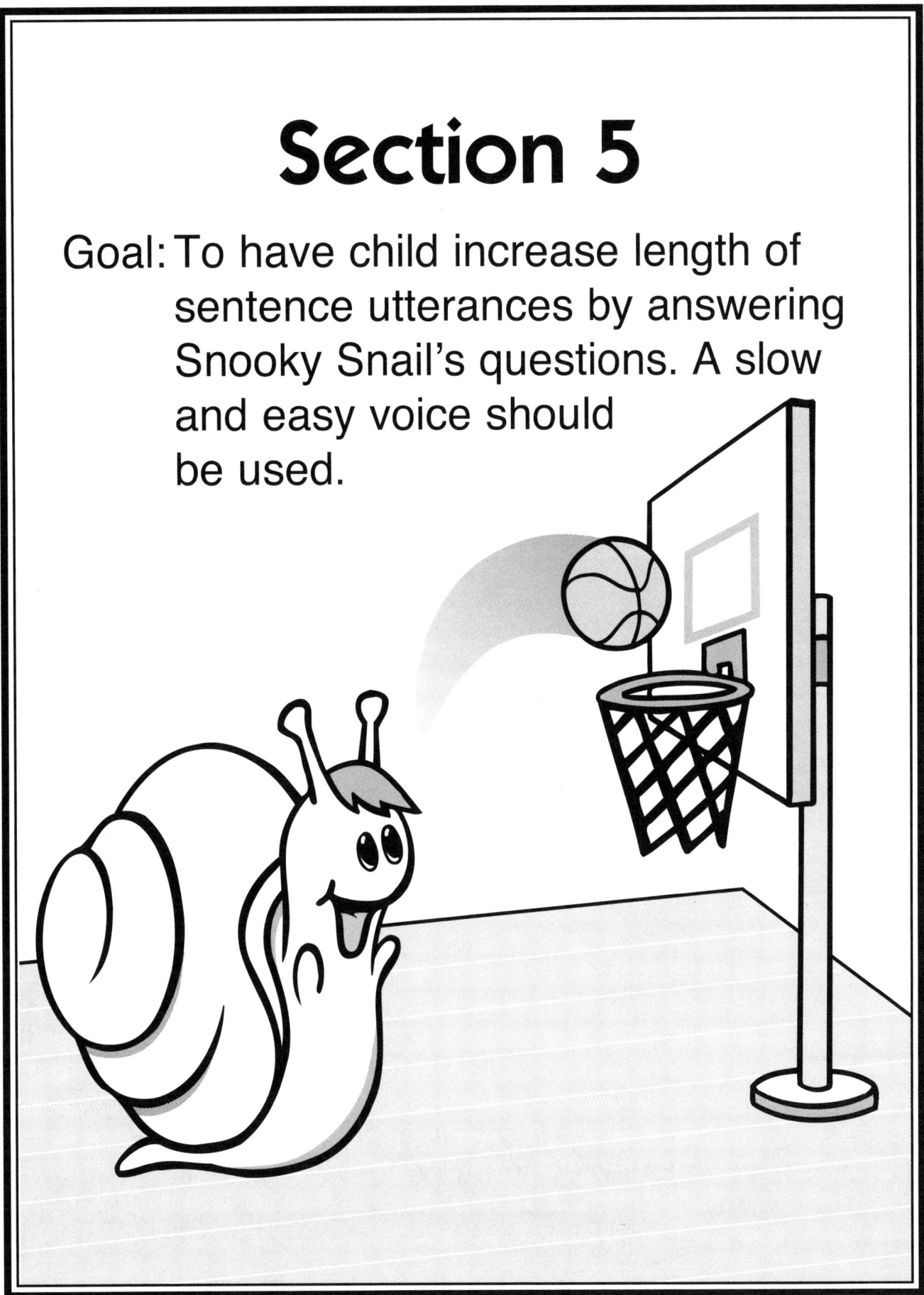

Draw a picture of your Mom. (You may also color, cut and paste pictures from page 81.) Describe her to Snooky using your slow and easy voice. "My Mom has _____."

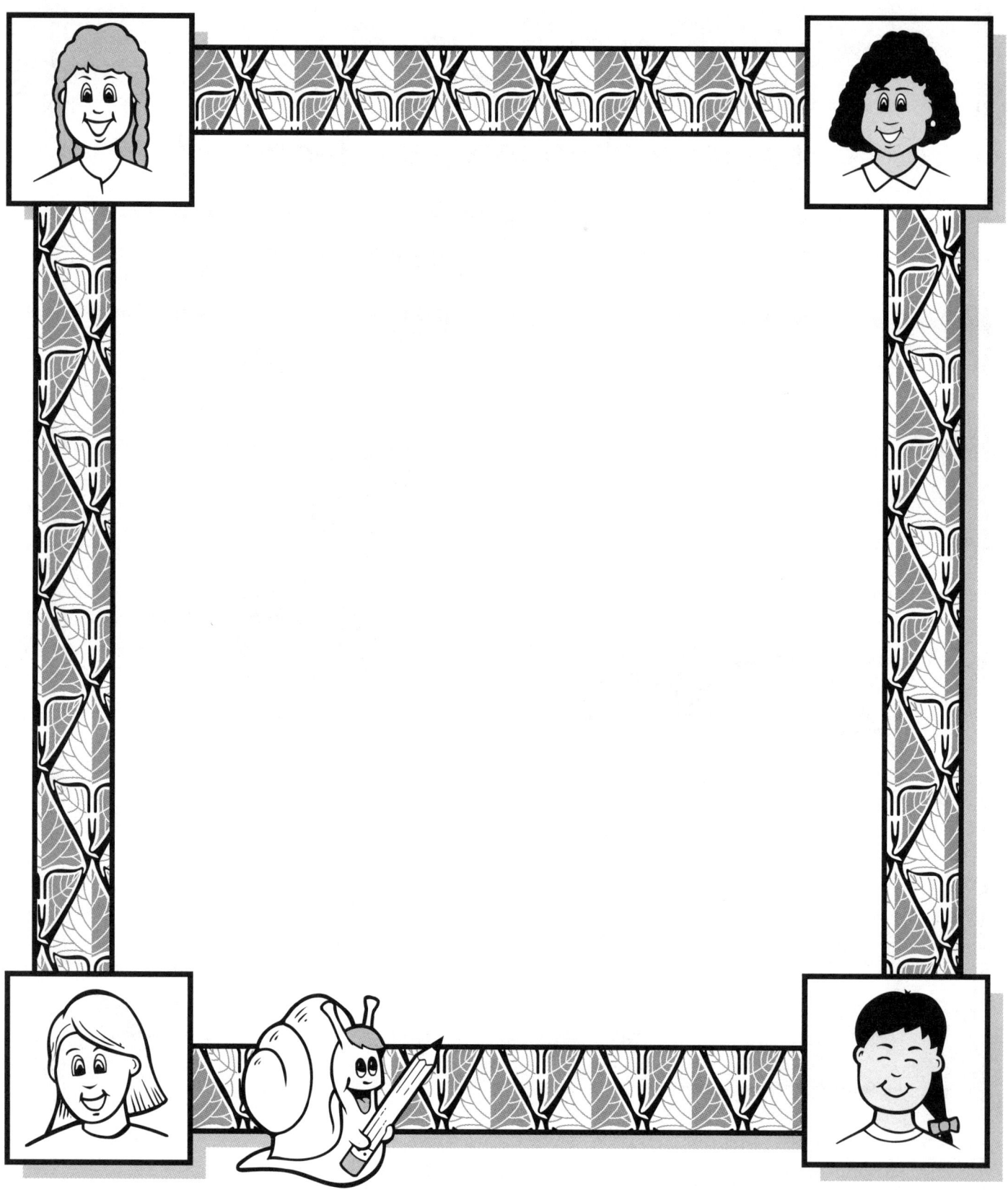

Draw a picture of your Dad. (You may also color, cut and paste pictures from page 81.) Describe him to Snooky using your slow and easy voice. "My Dad has _____."

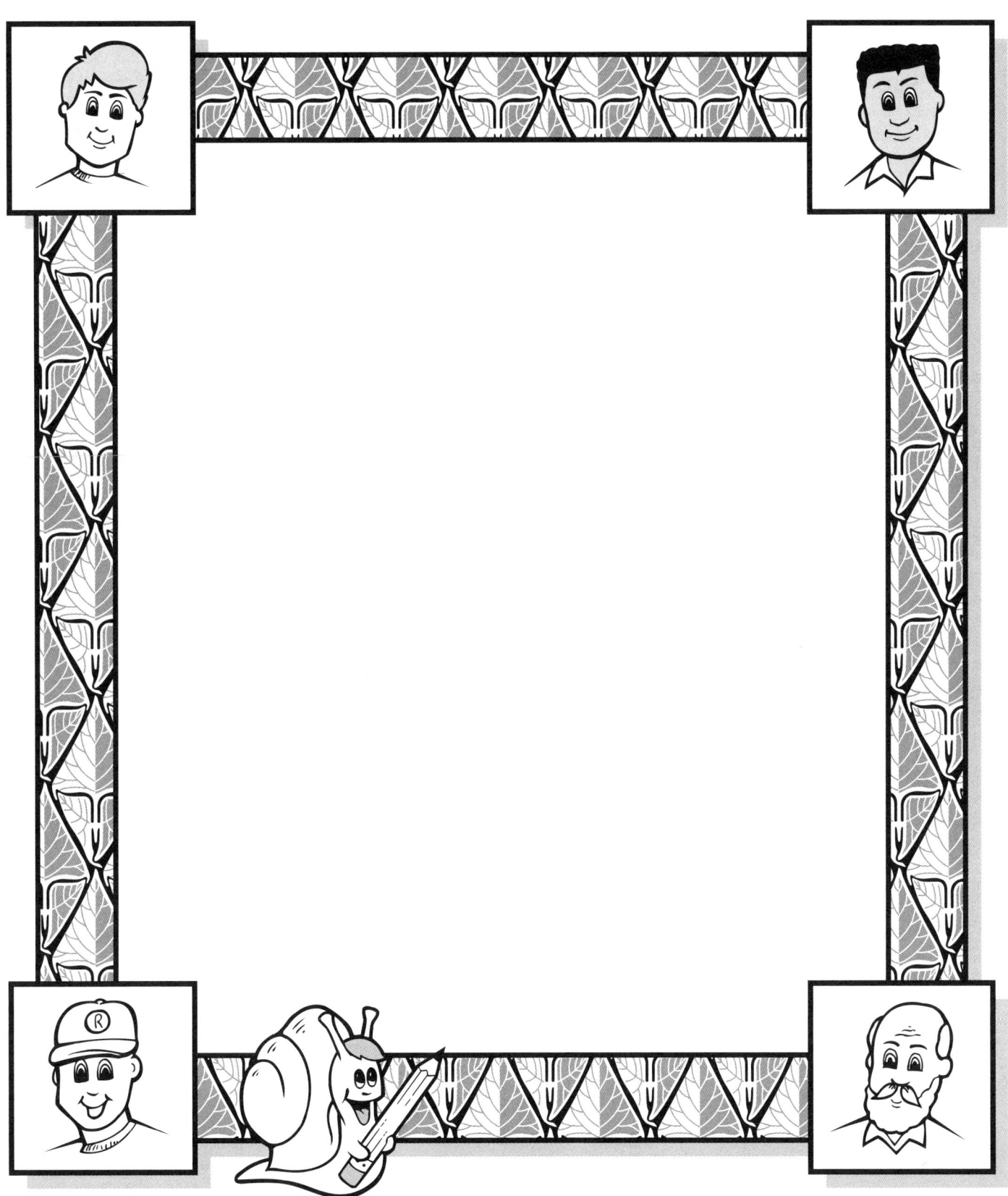

Name   Date   Helper's Signature

Draw a picture of your bedroom. (You may also color, cut and paste pictures from page 77.) Describe it to Snooky using your slow and easy voice. "My bedroom has _____."

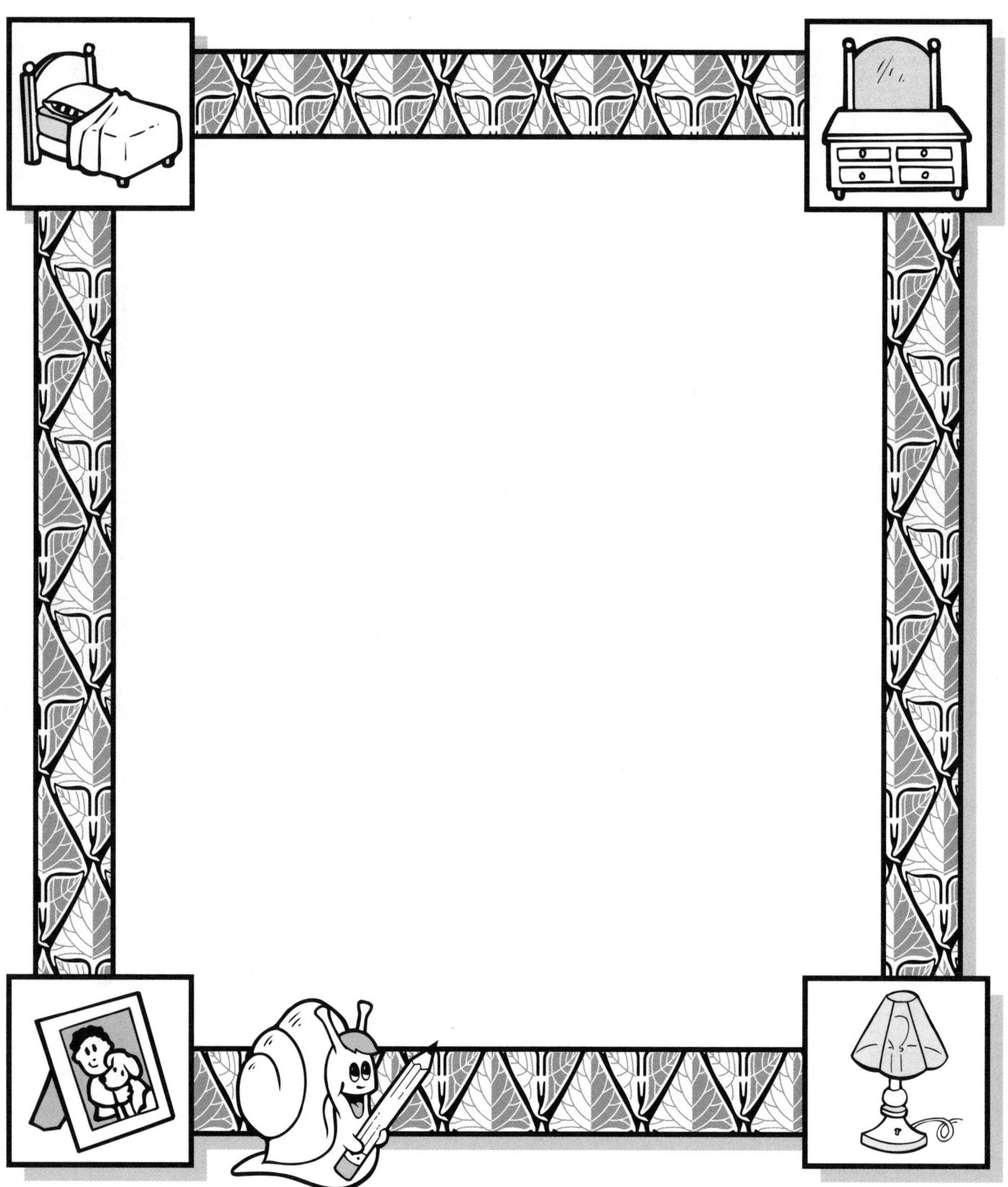

Draw a picture of your pet. (You may also color, cut and paste pictures from pages 82 and 91.) Describe it to Snooky using your slow and easy voice. "My pet has _____."

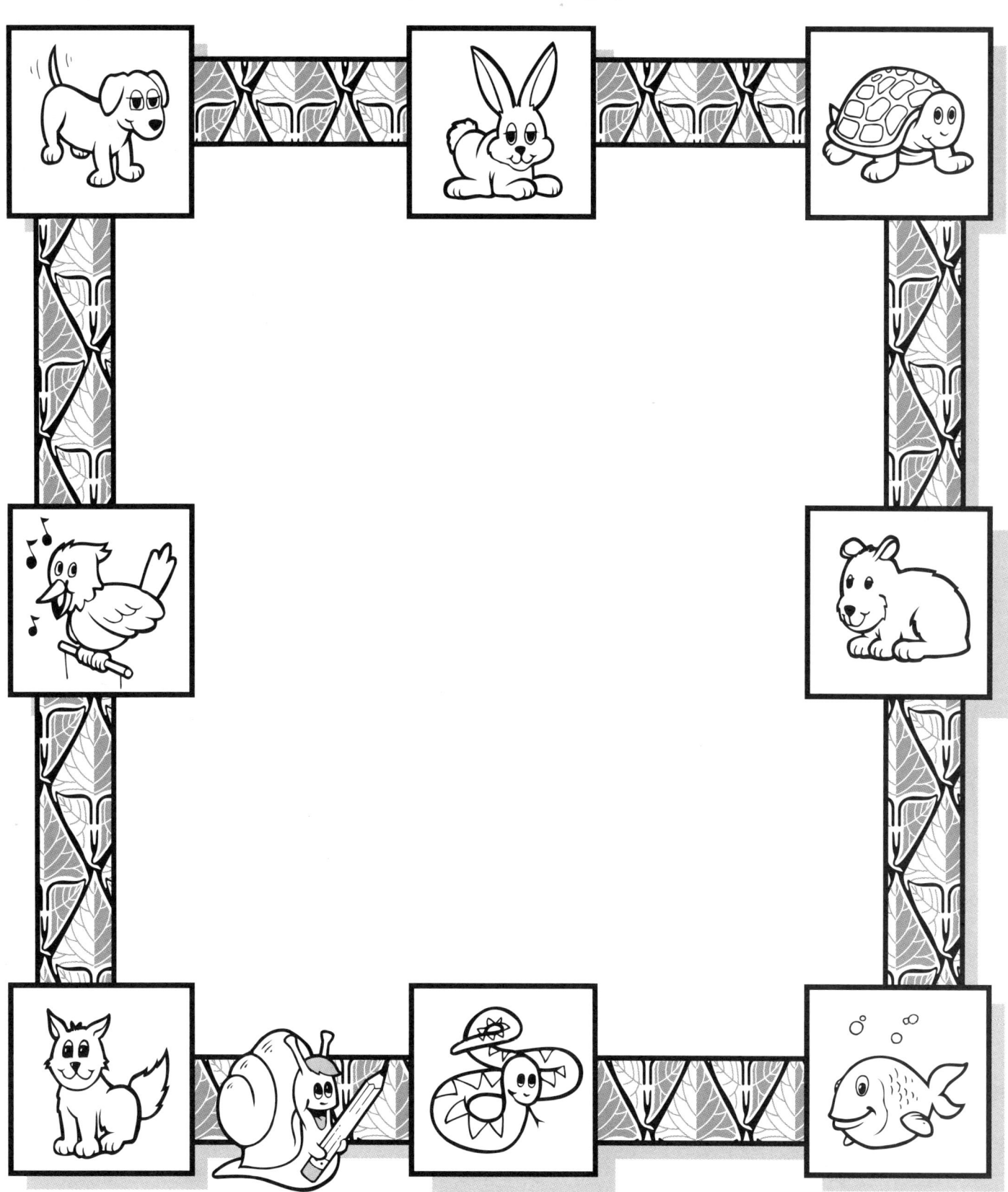

Name _____ Date _____ Helper's Signature _____

Draw a picture of your playground. (You may also color, cut and paste pictures from page 87.) Describe it to Snooky using your slow and easy voice. "My playground has _____."

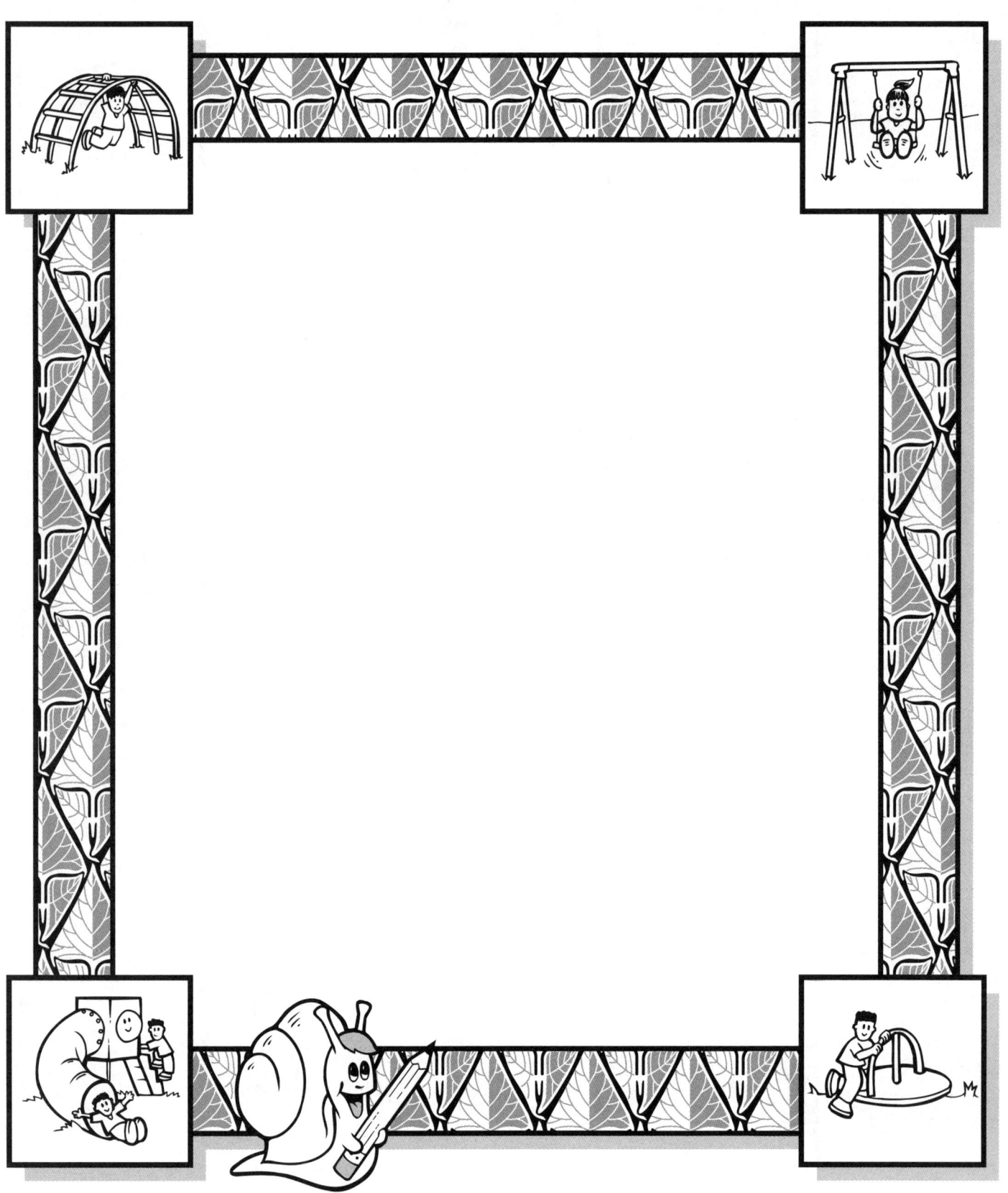

Draw a picture of something you don't like to eat. (You may also color, cut and paste pictures from pages 83-85.) Describe it to Snooky using your slow and easy voice. "I don't like to eat _____."

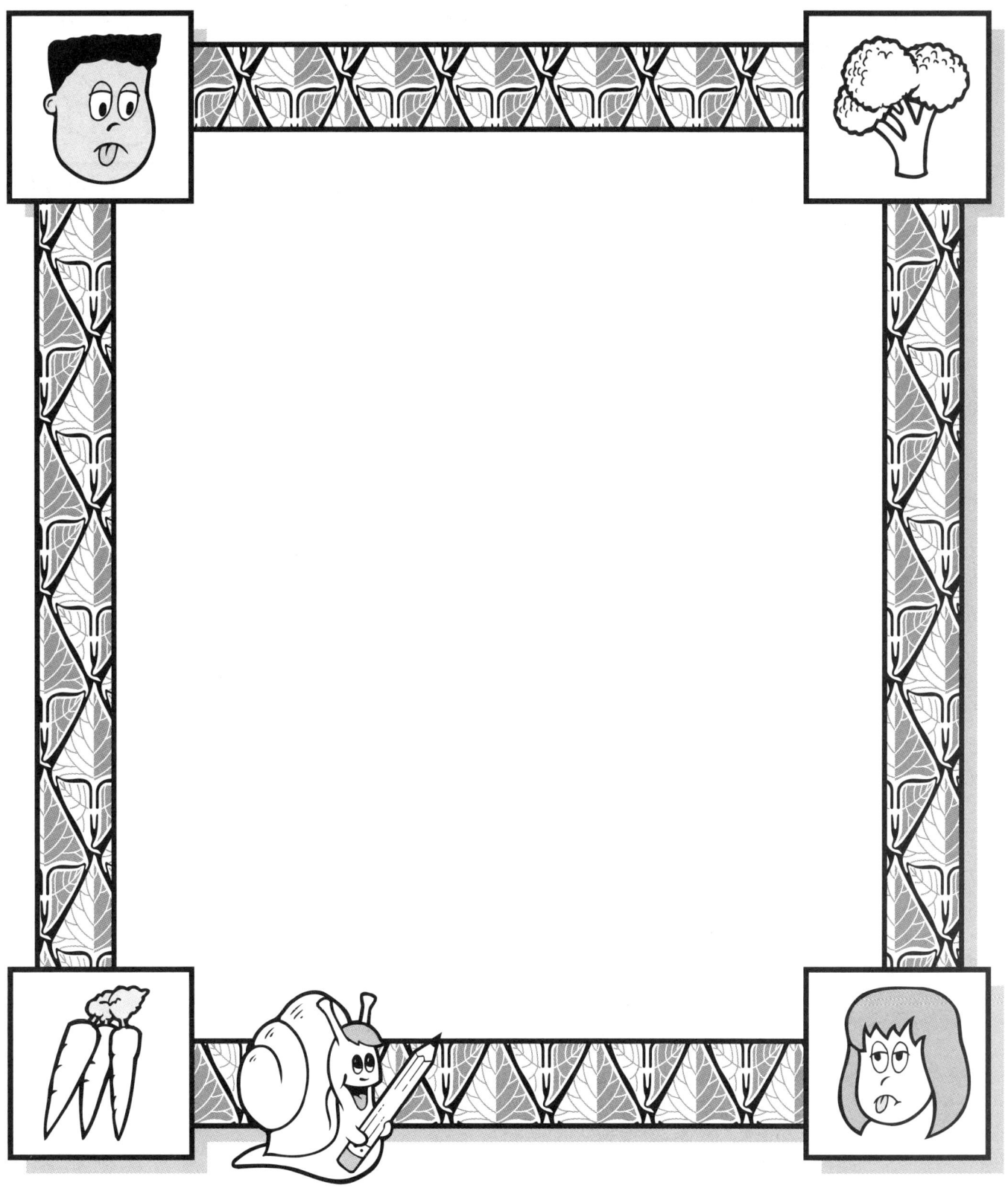

Draw a picture of something you like to wear. (You may also color, cut and paste pictures from page 80.) Describe it to Snooky using your slow and easy voice. "I like to wear _____."

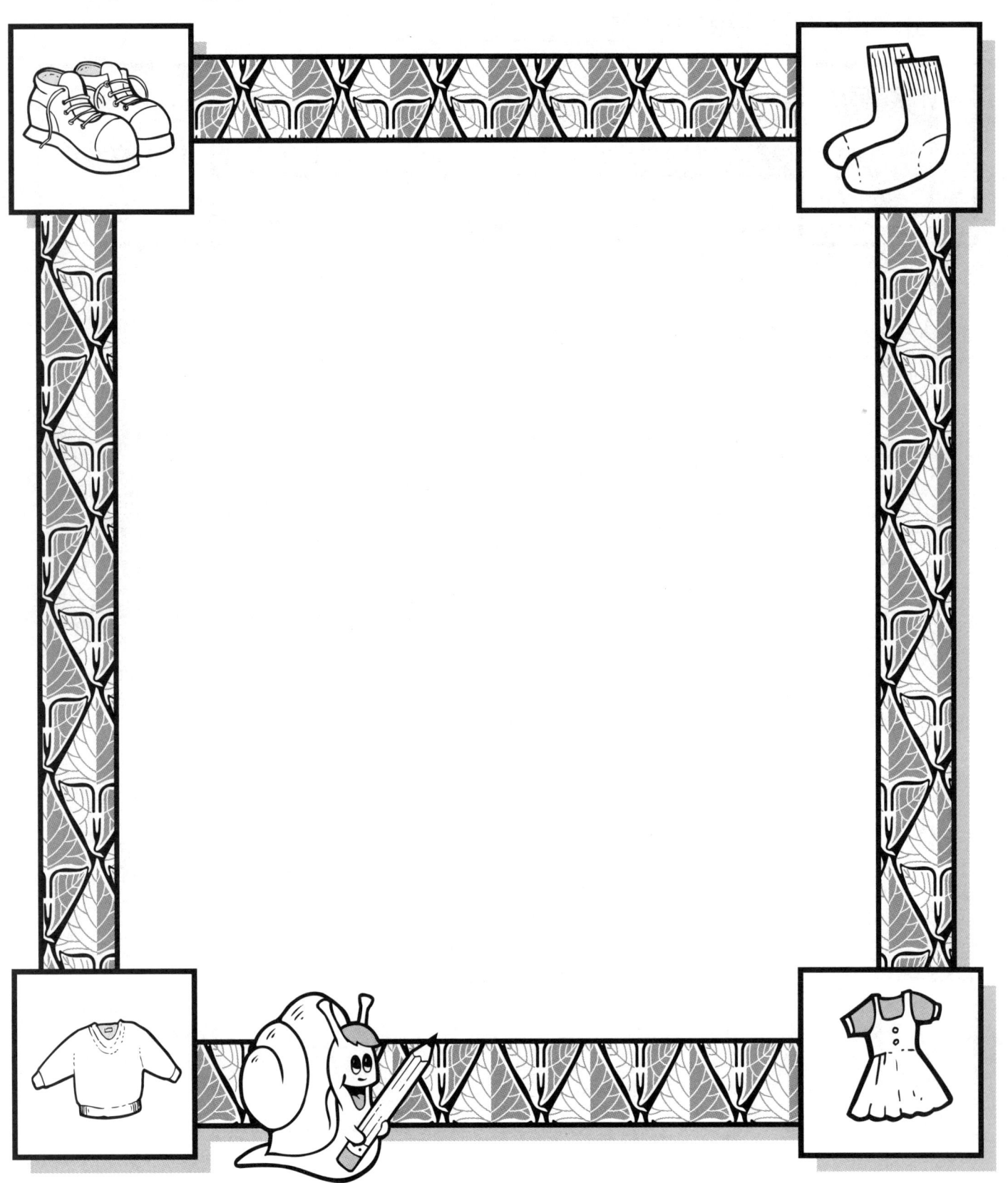

Draw a picture of what you saw at the circus. (You may also color, cut and paste pictures from page 79.) Describe it to Snooky using your slow and easy voice. "At the circus I saw _____."

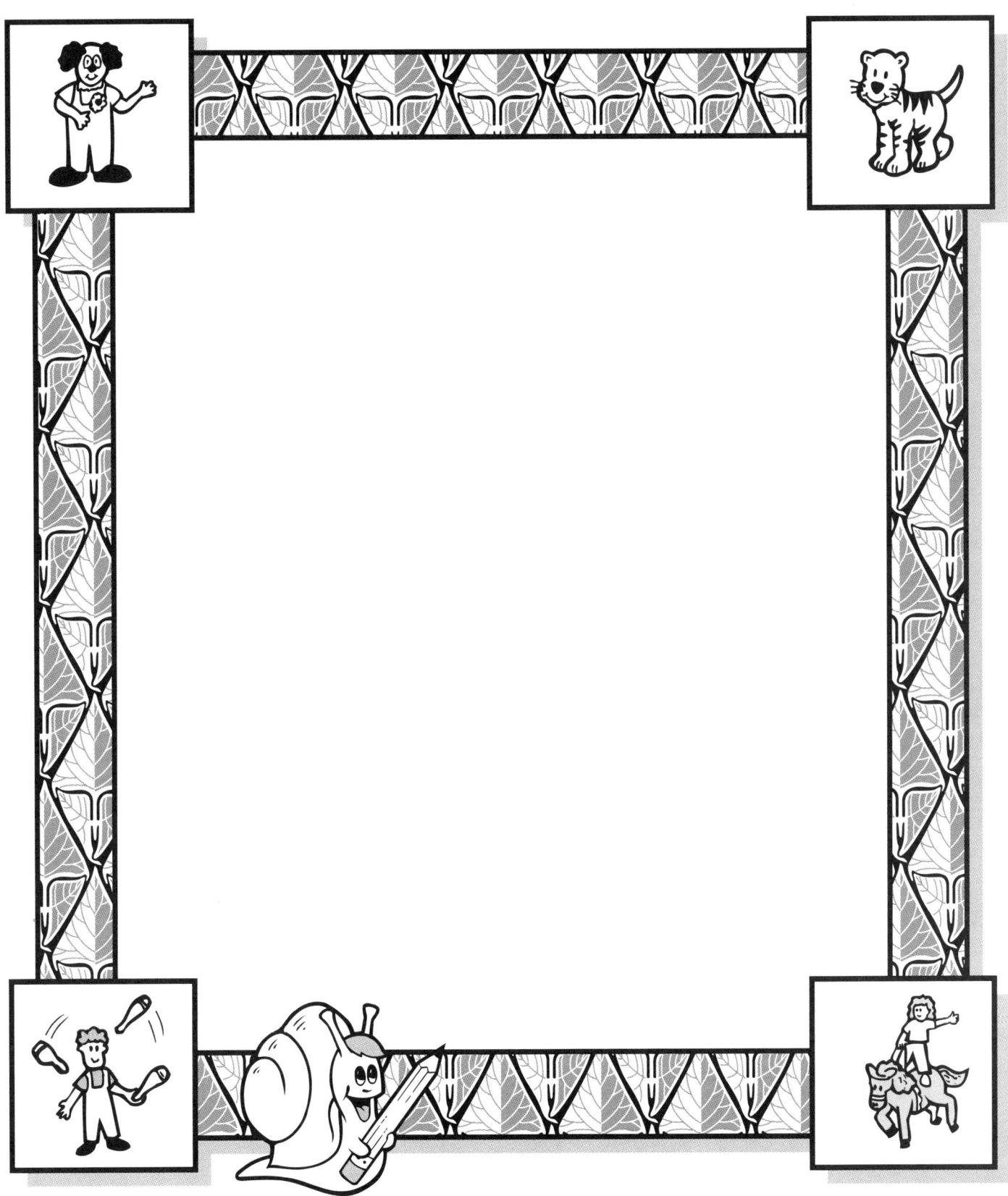

Name　　　　　　　Date　　　　Helper's Signature

Draw a picture of what you saw at the beach. (You may also color, cut and paste pictures from page 76.) Describe it to Snooky using your slow and easy voice. "At the beach I saw _____."

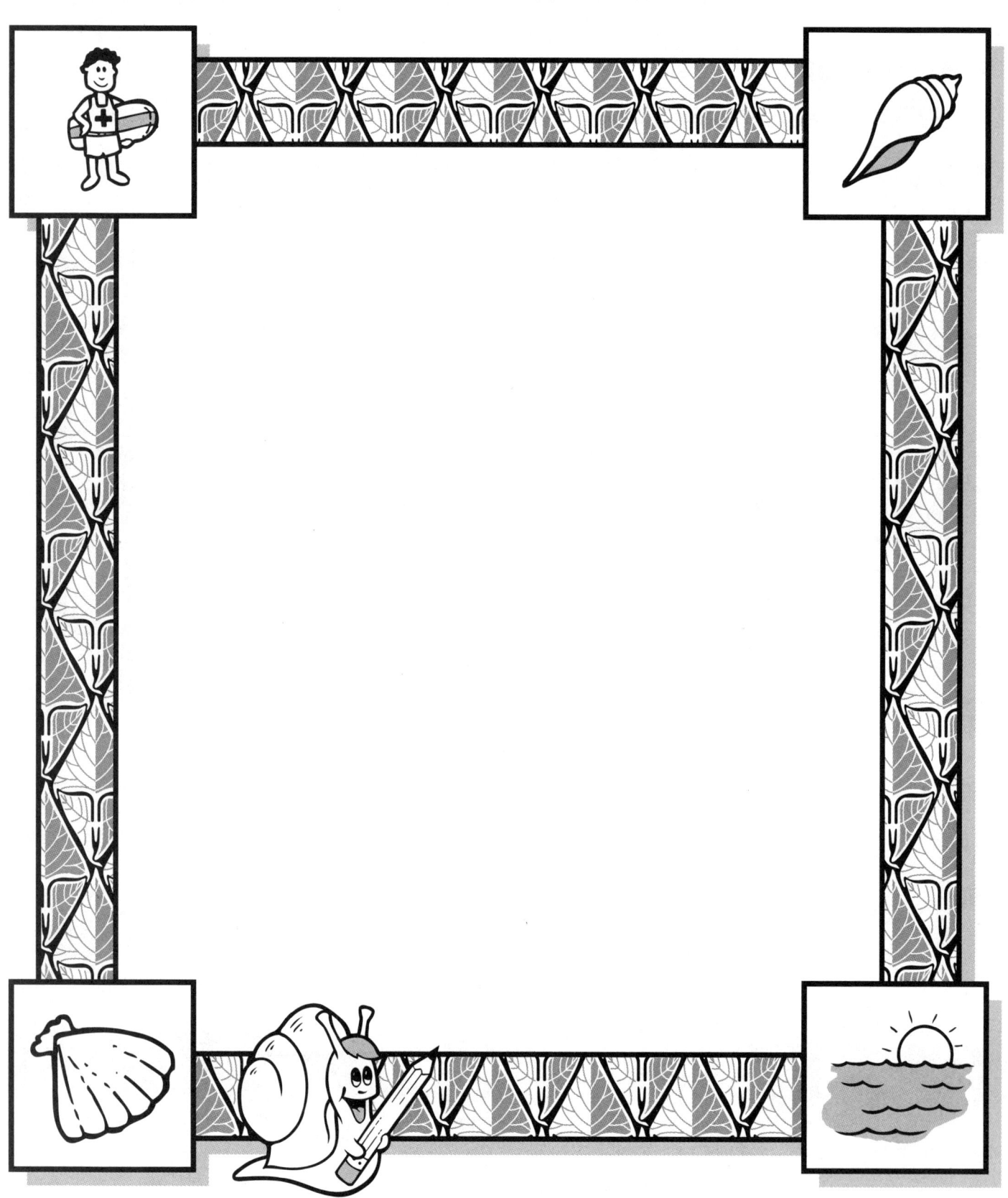

Draw a picture of what you saw at the grocery store. (You may also color, cut and paste pictures from pages 83-86.) Describe it to Snooky using your slow and easy voice. "At the grocery store I saw _____."

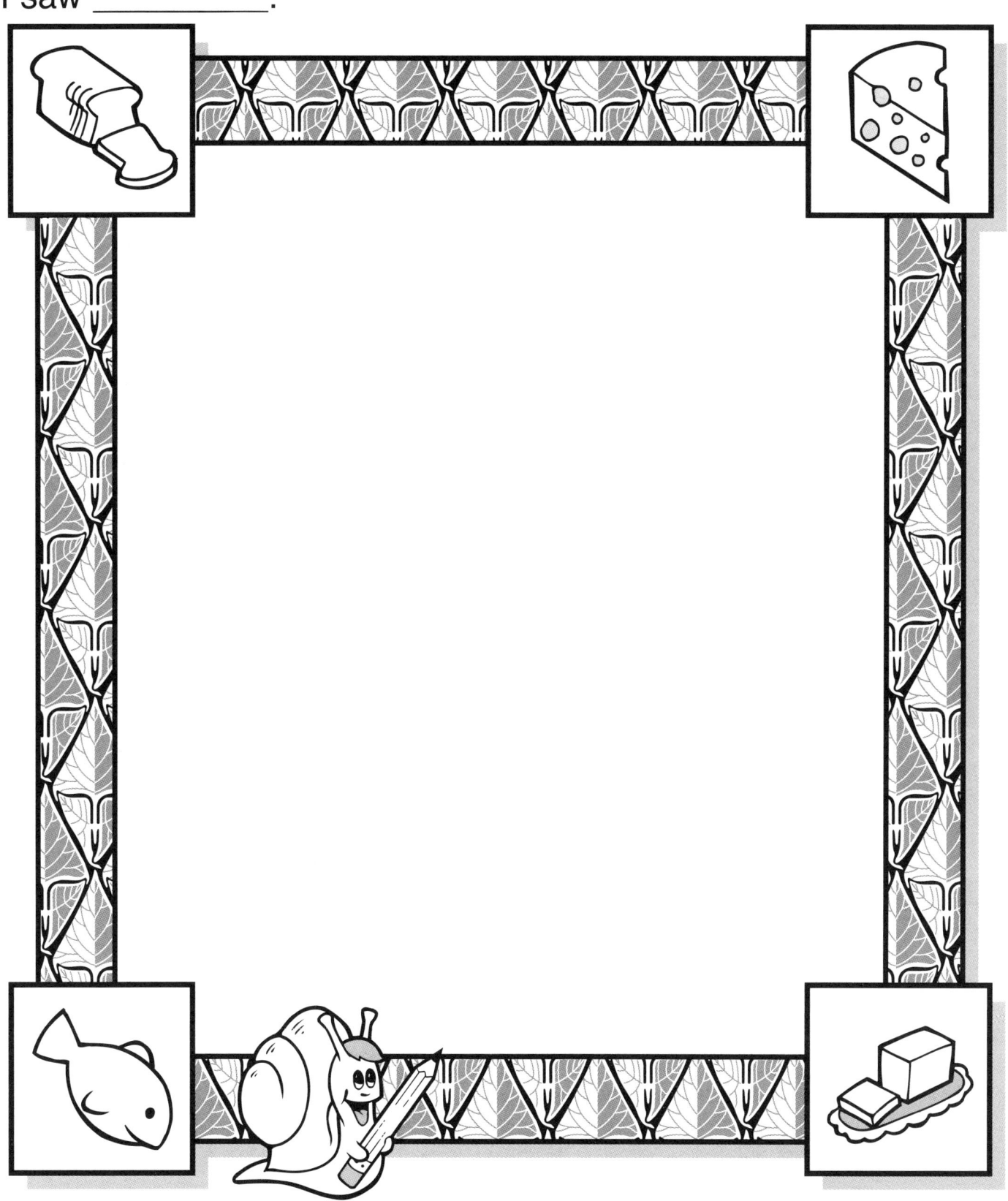

Draw a picture of what you saw at the toy store. (You may also color, cut and paste pictures from page 87.) Describe it to Snooky using your slow and easy voice. "At the toy store I saw _____."

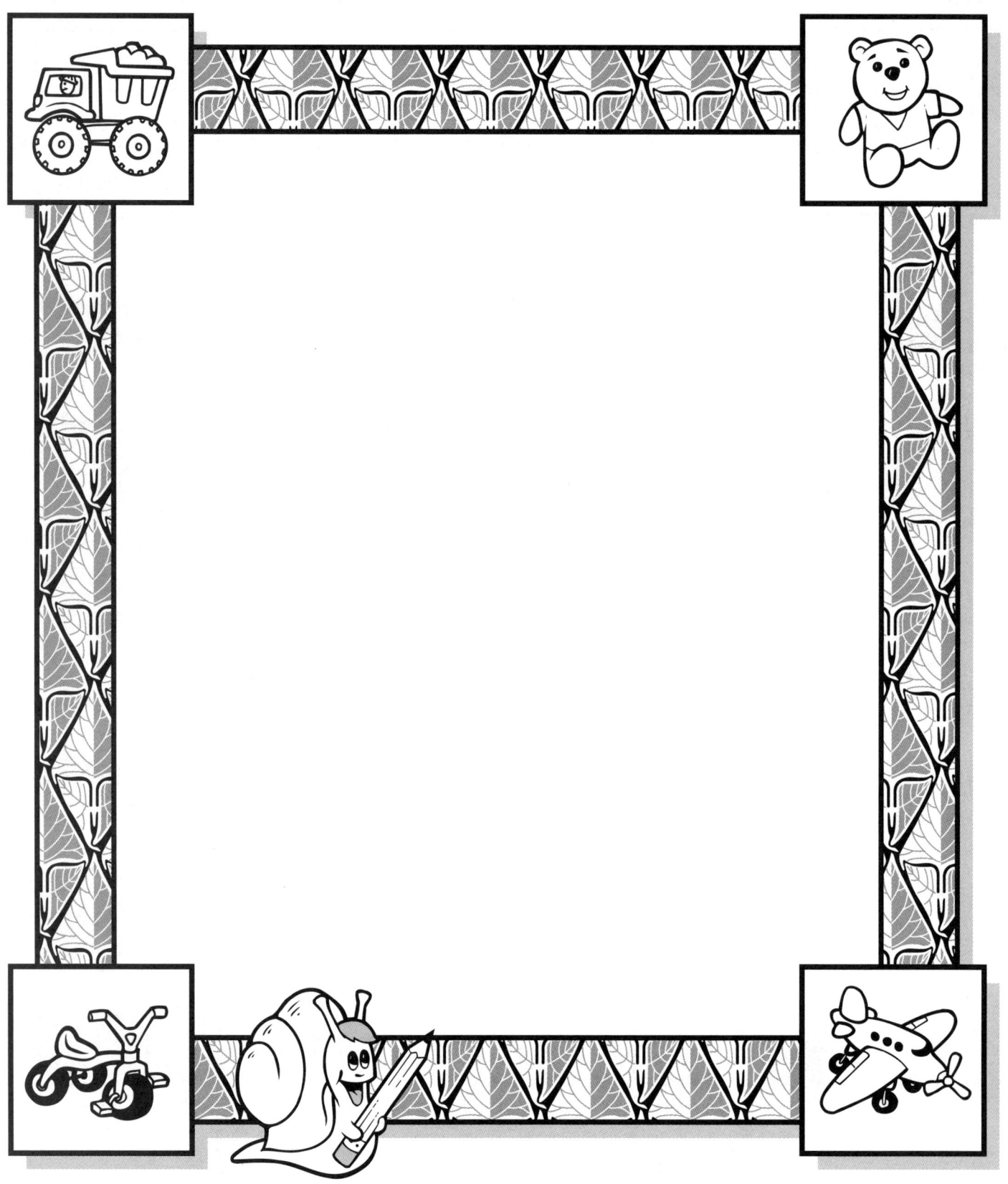

Section 6

Goal: To have child spontaneously use a slow and easy voice while describing various scenes involving Snooky Snail.

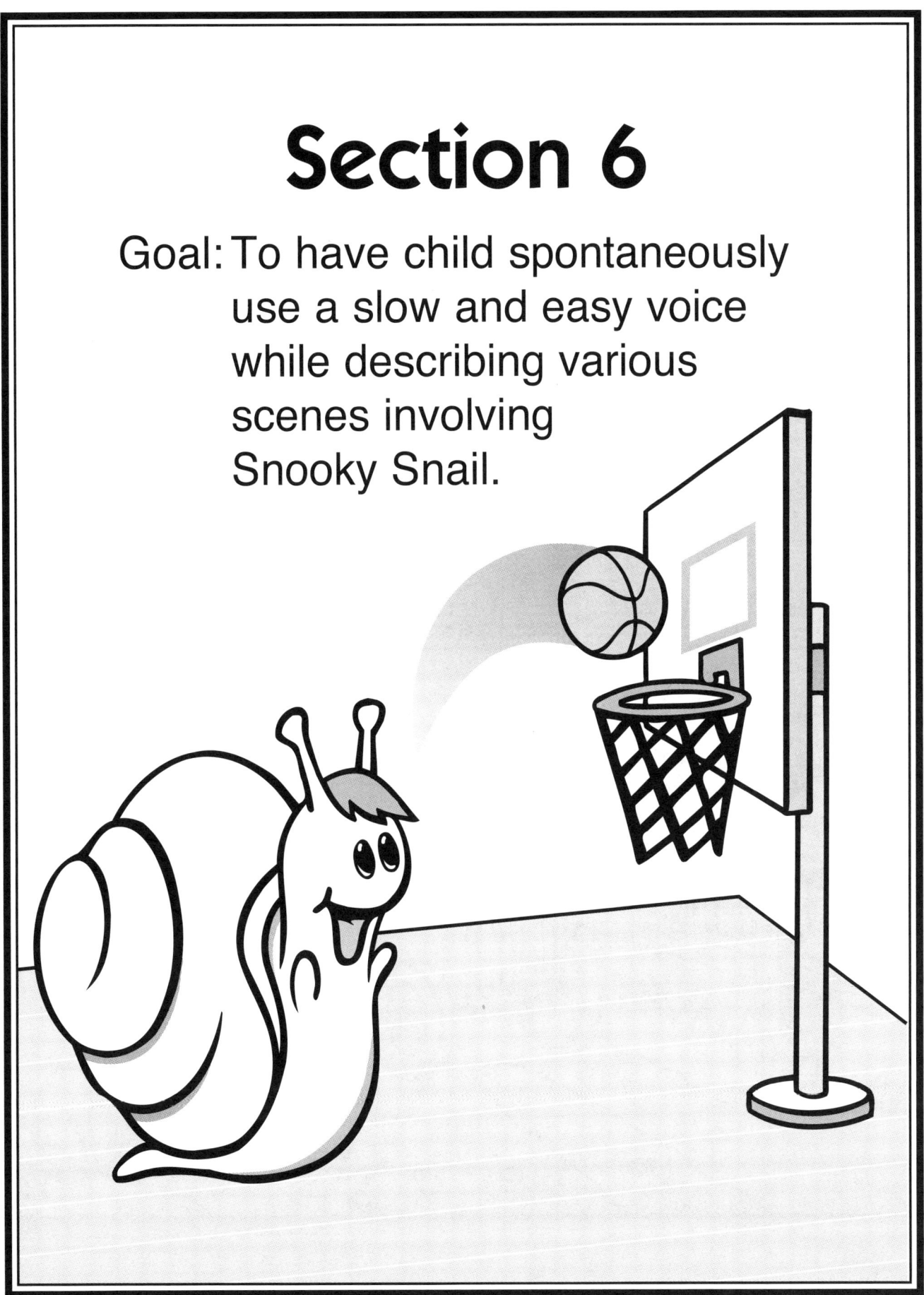

Snooky is hiding on the farm! Can you find and circle him in six different places? Tell where he is using your slow and easy voice.

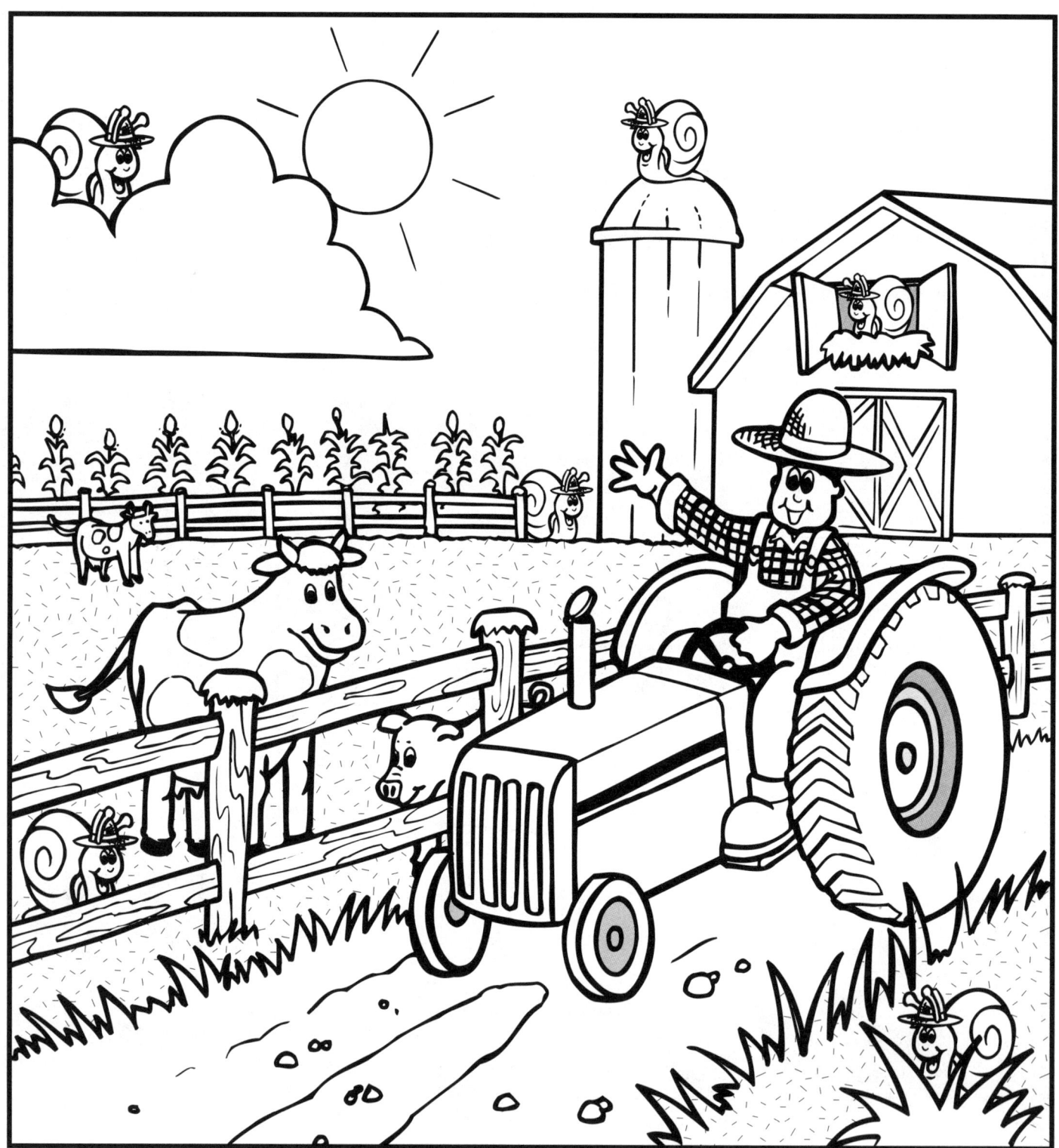

Snooky is hiding in the playground! Can you find and circle him in six different places? Tell where he is using your slow and easy voice.

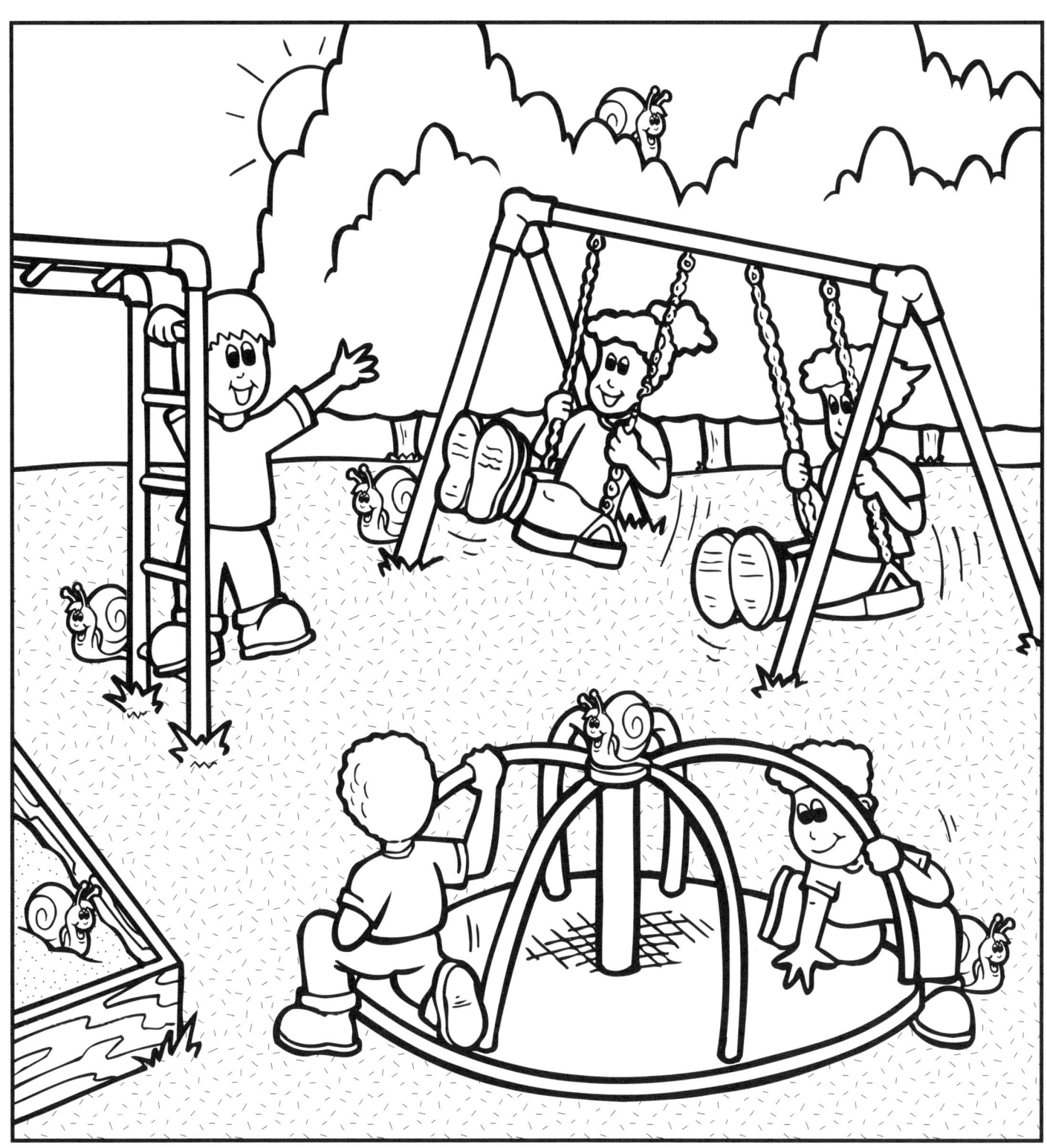

Snooky is hiding at school! Can you find and circle him in six different places? Tell where he is using your slow and easy voice.

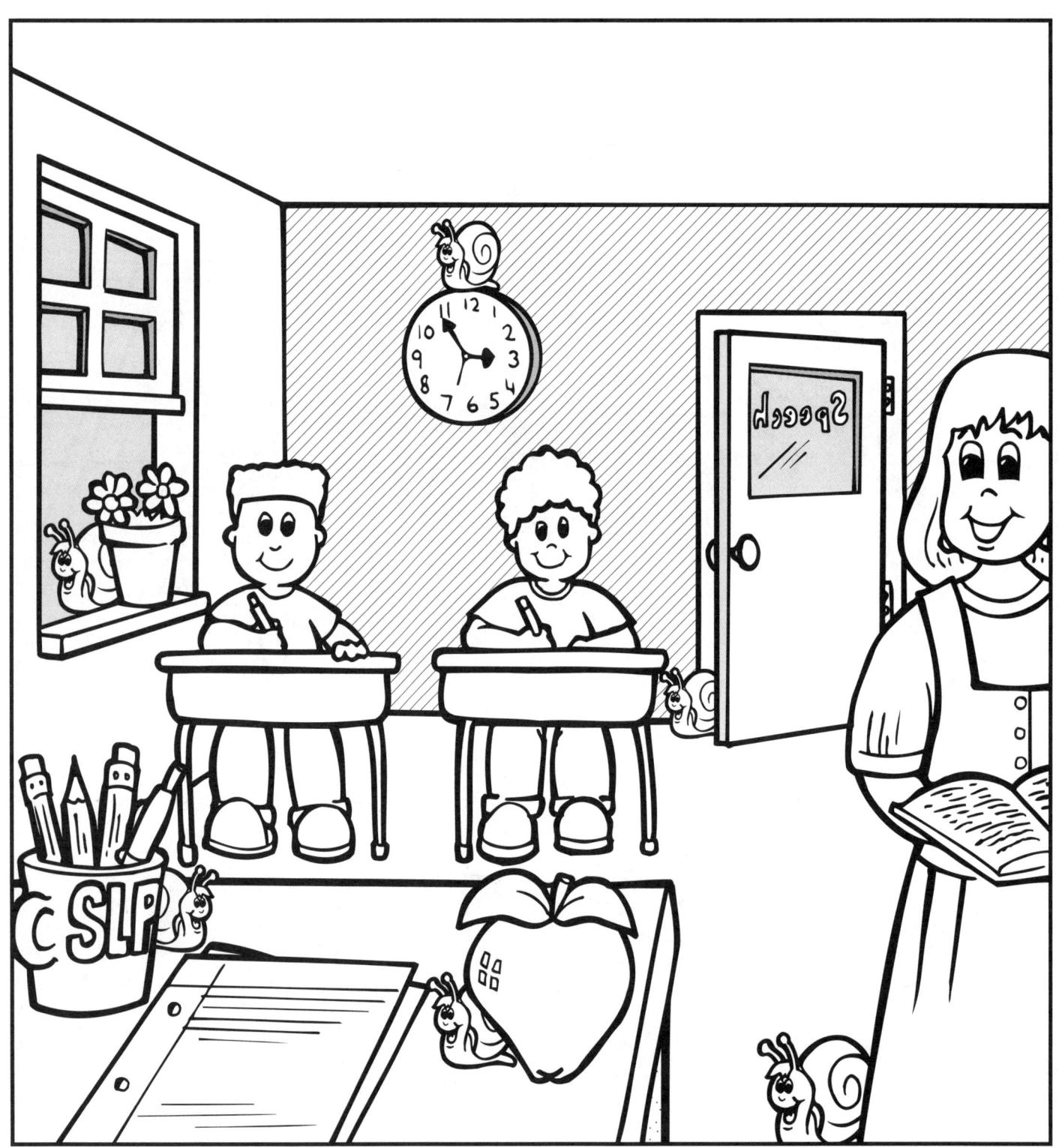

Snooky is hiding at the zoo! Can you find and circle him in six different places? Tell where he is using your slow and easy voice.

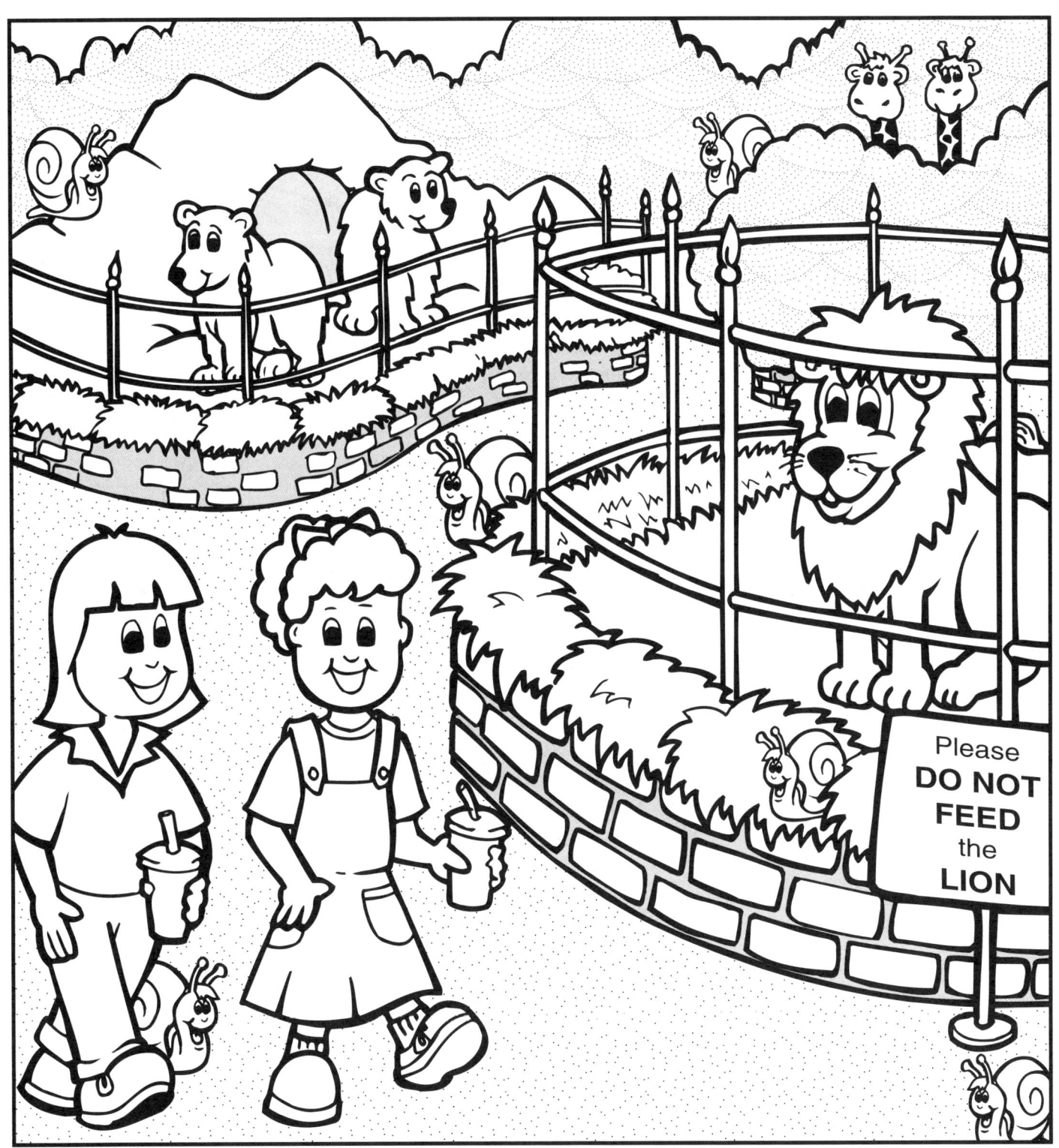

Snooky is hiding at the birthday party! Can you find and circle him in six different places? Tell where he is using your slow and easy voice.

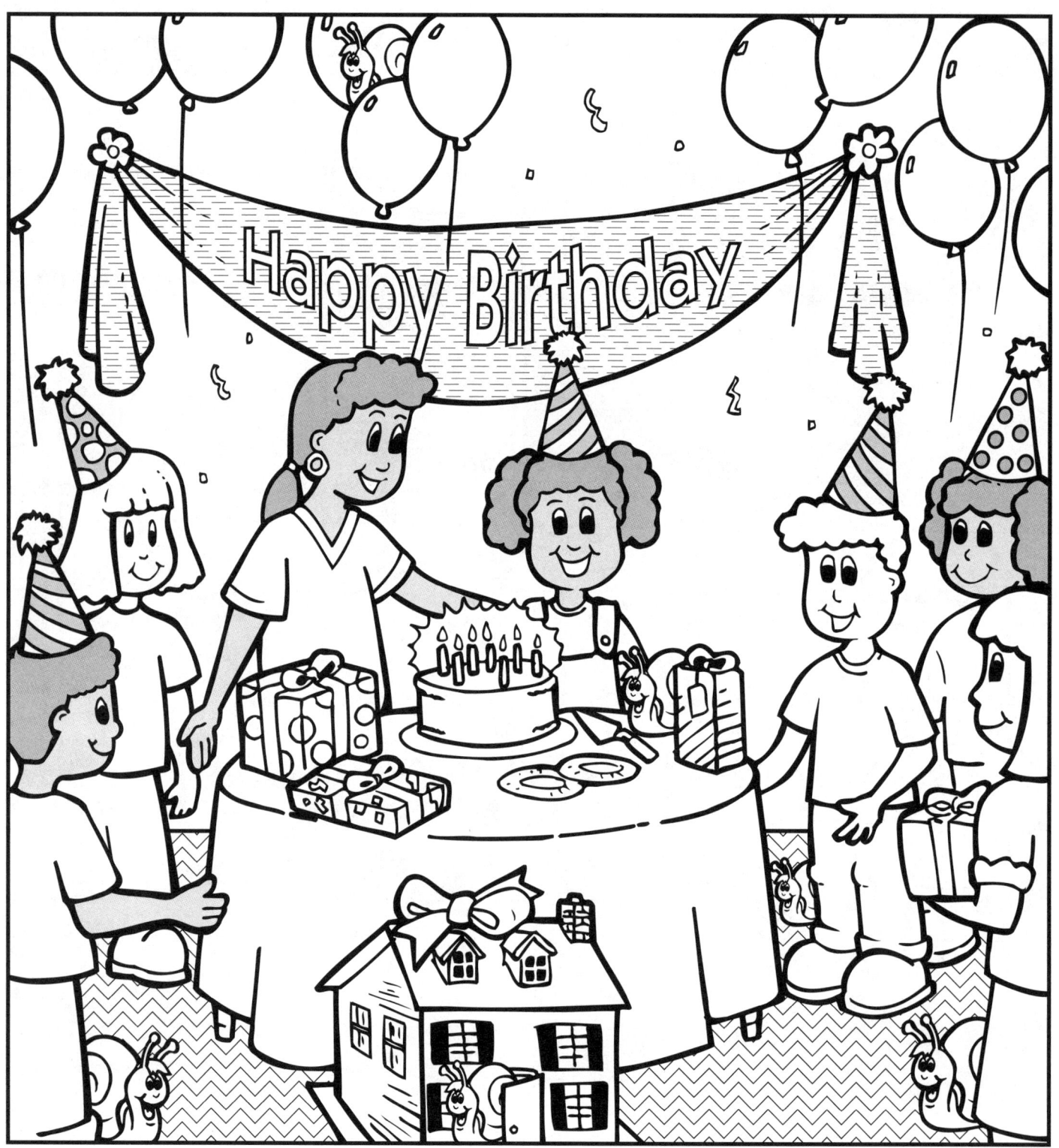

Snooky is hiding at the beach! Can you find and circle him in six different places? Tell where he is using your slow and easy voice.

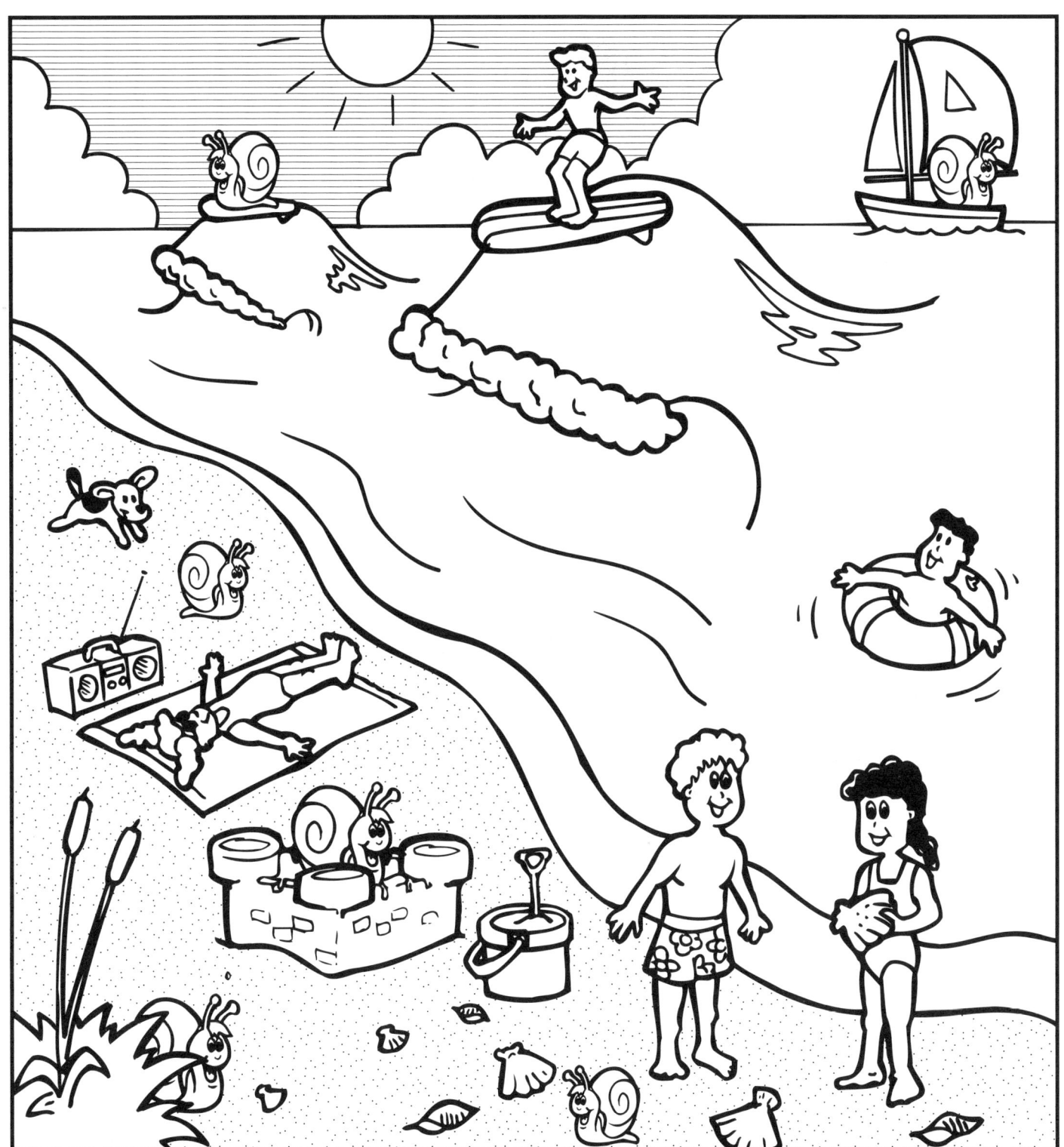

Snooky is hiding at the picnic! Can you find and circle him in six different places? Tell where he is using your slow and easy voice.

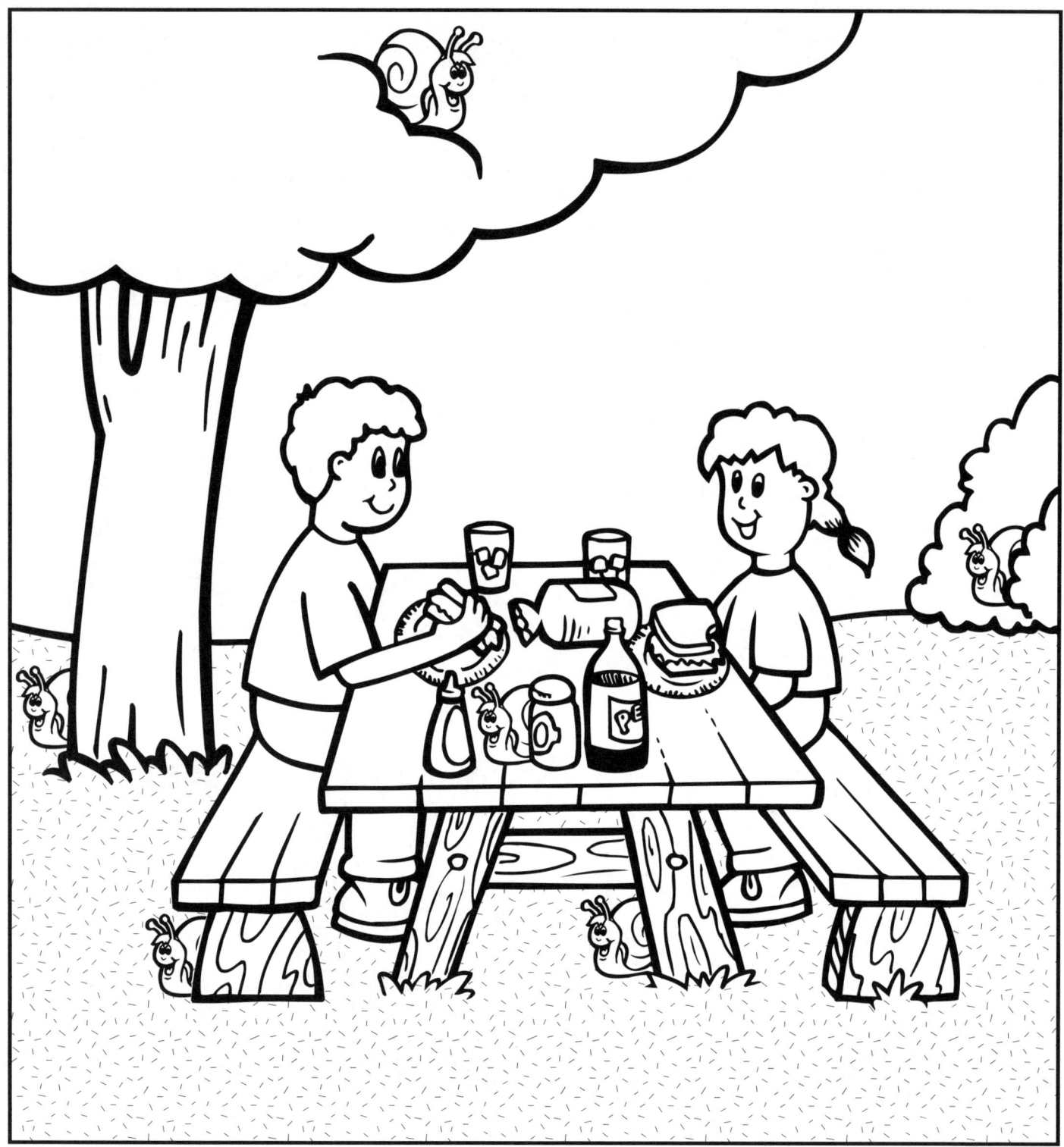

Snooky is hiding at the Halloween Party! Can you find and circle him in six different places? Tell where he is using your slow and easy voice.

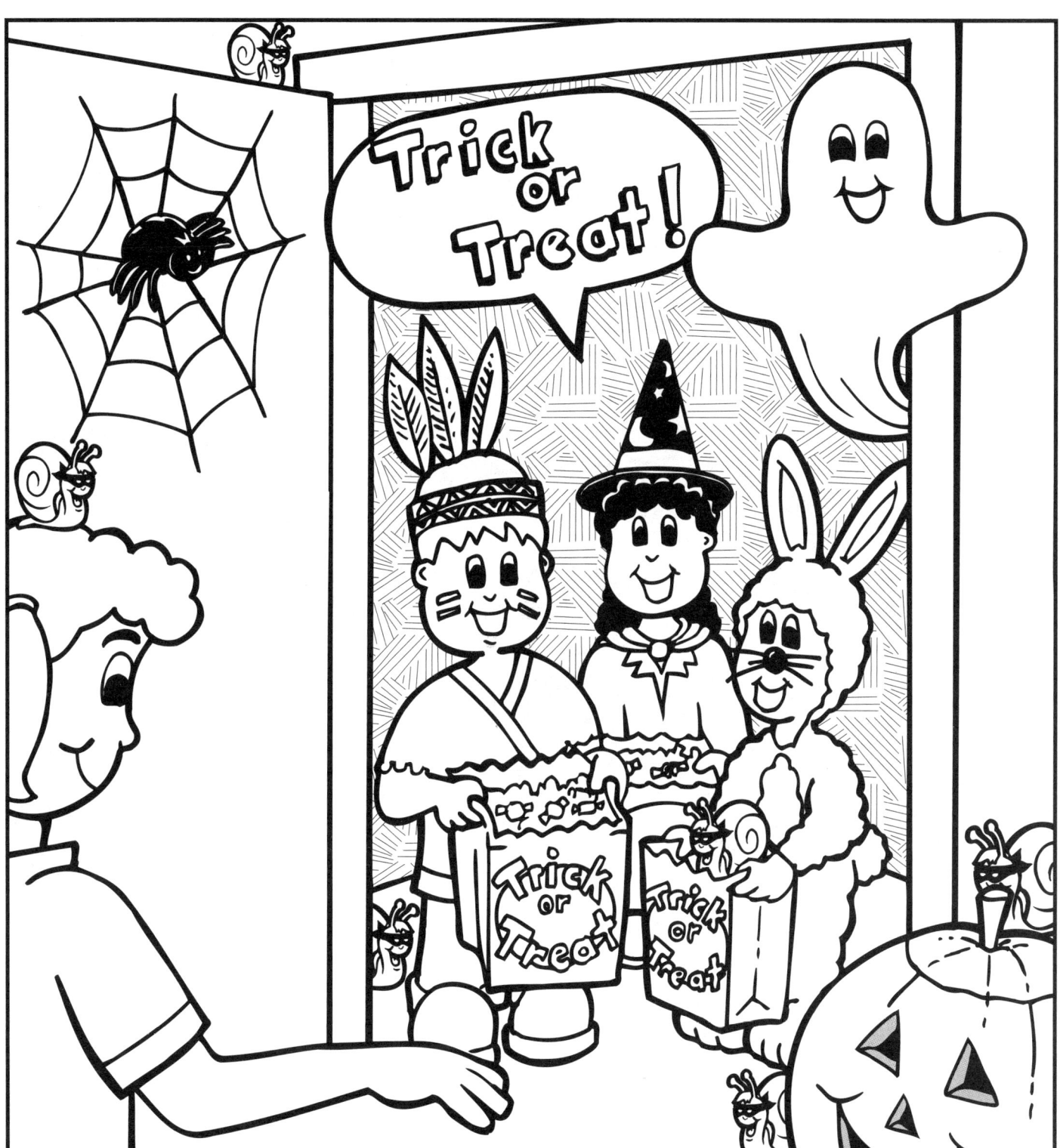

Snooky is hiding in the winter scene! Can you find and circle him in six different places? Tell where he is using your slow and easy voice.

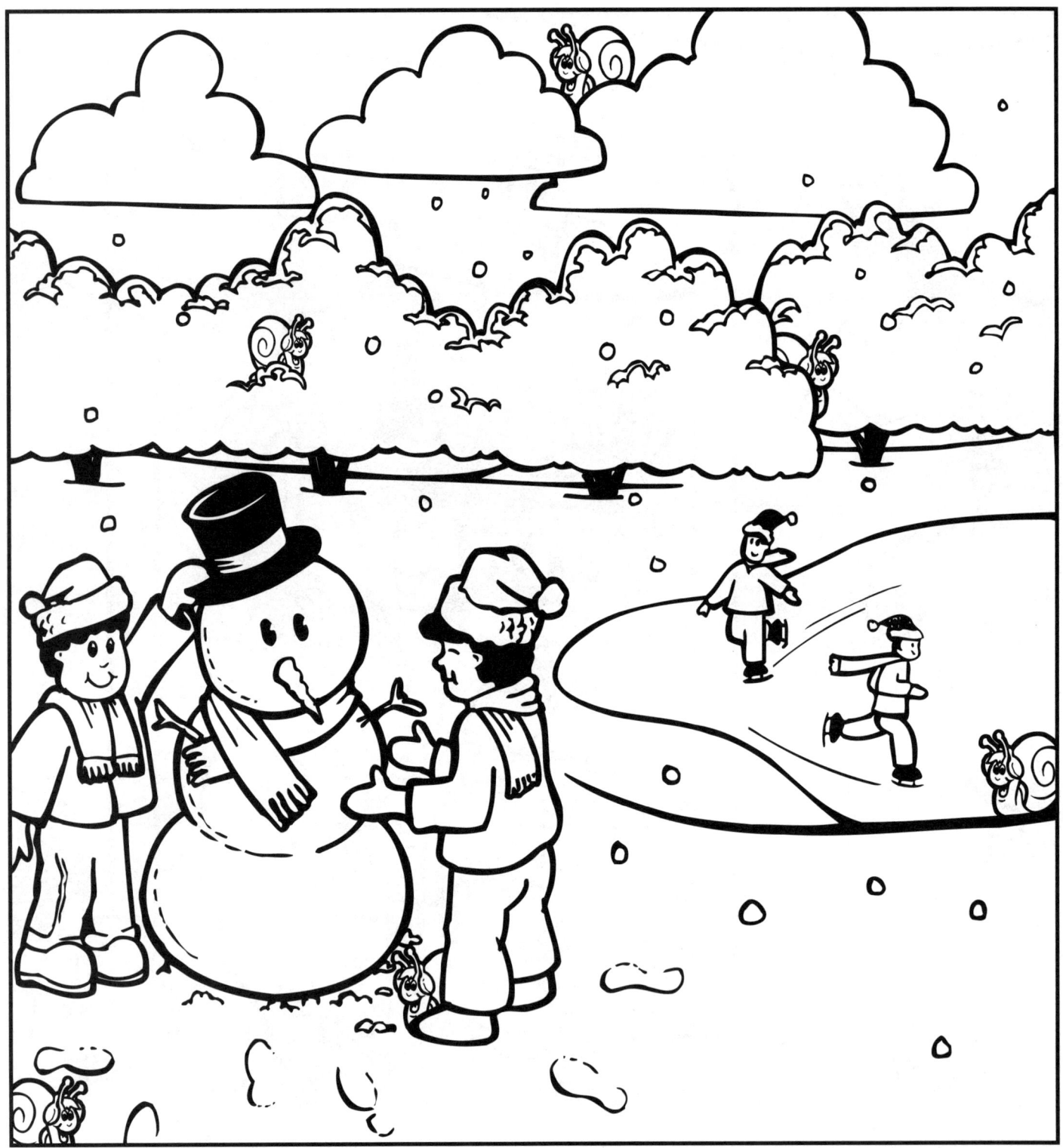

Snooky is hiding in this Christmas scene! Can you find and circle him in six different places? Tell where he is using your slow and easy voice.

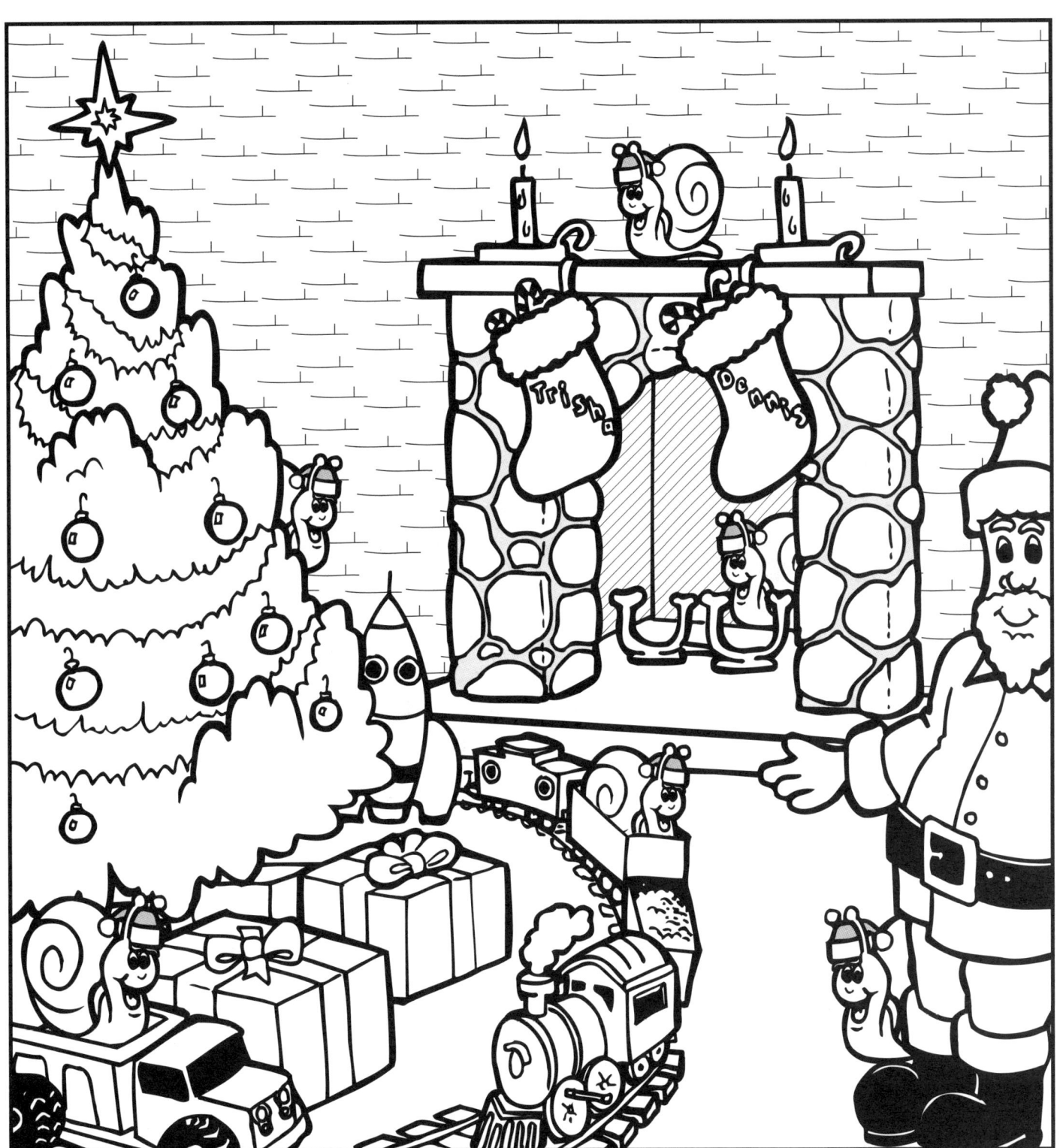

Snooky is hiding at the Easter egg hunt! Can you find and circle him in six different places? Tell where he is using your slow and easy voice.

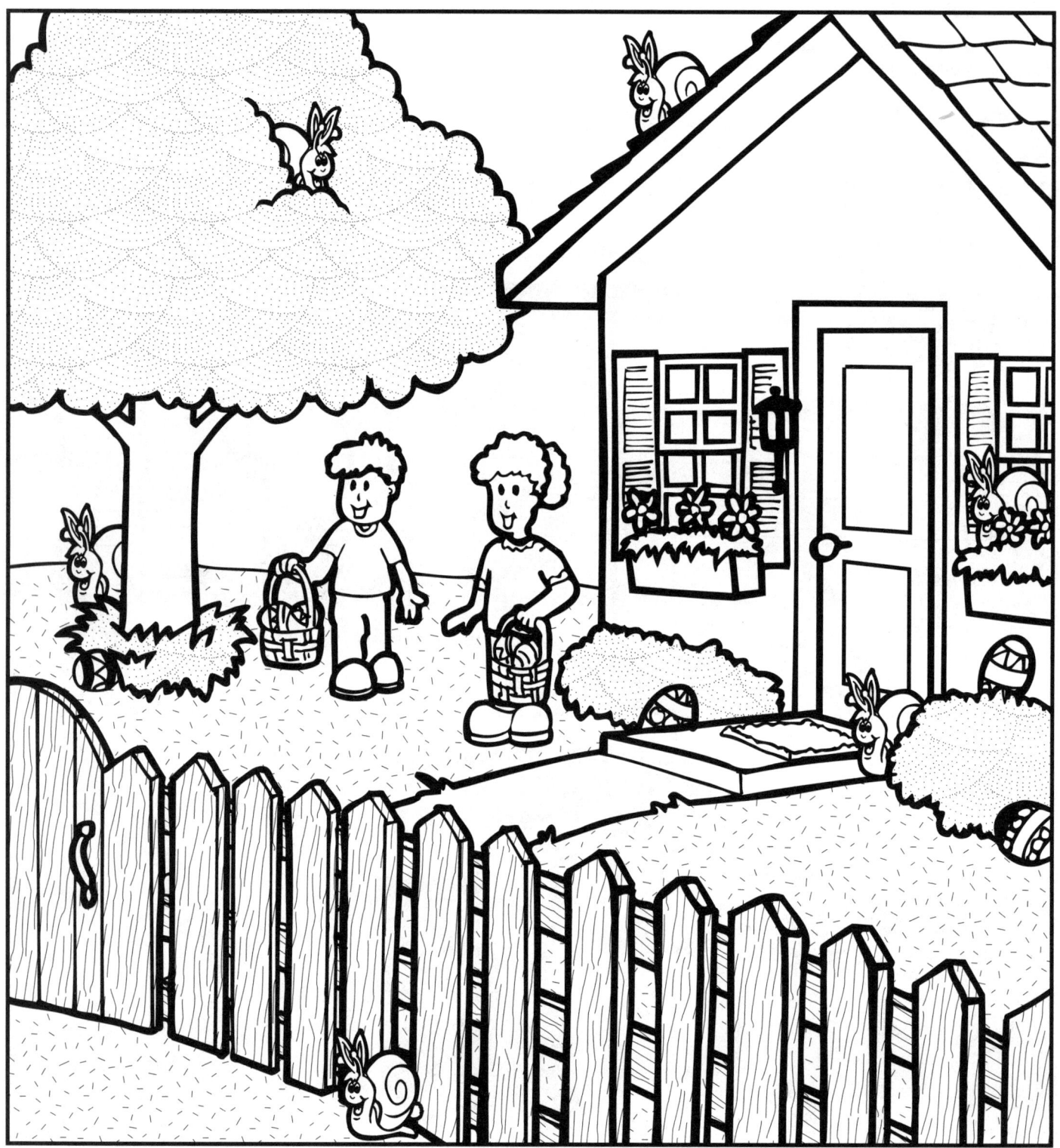

Section 7
Puppets and Scenes for Role-playing!

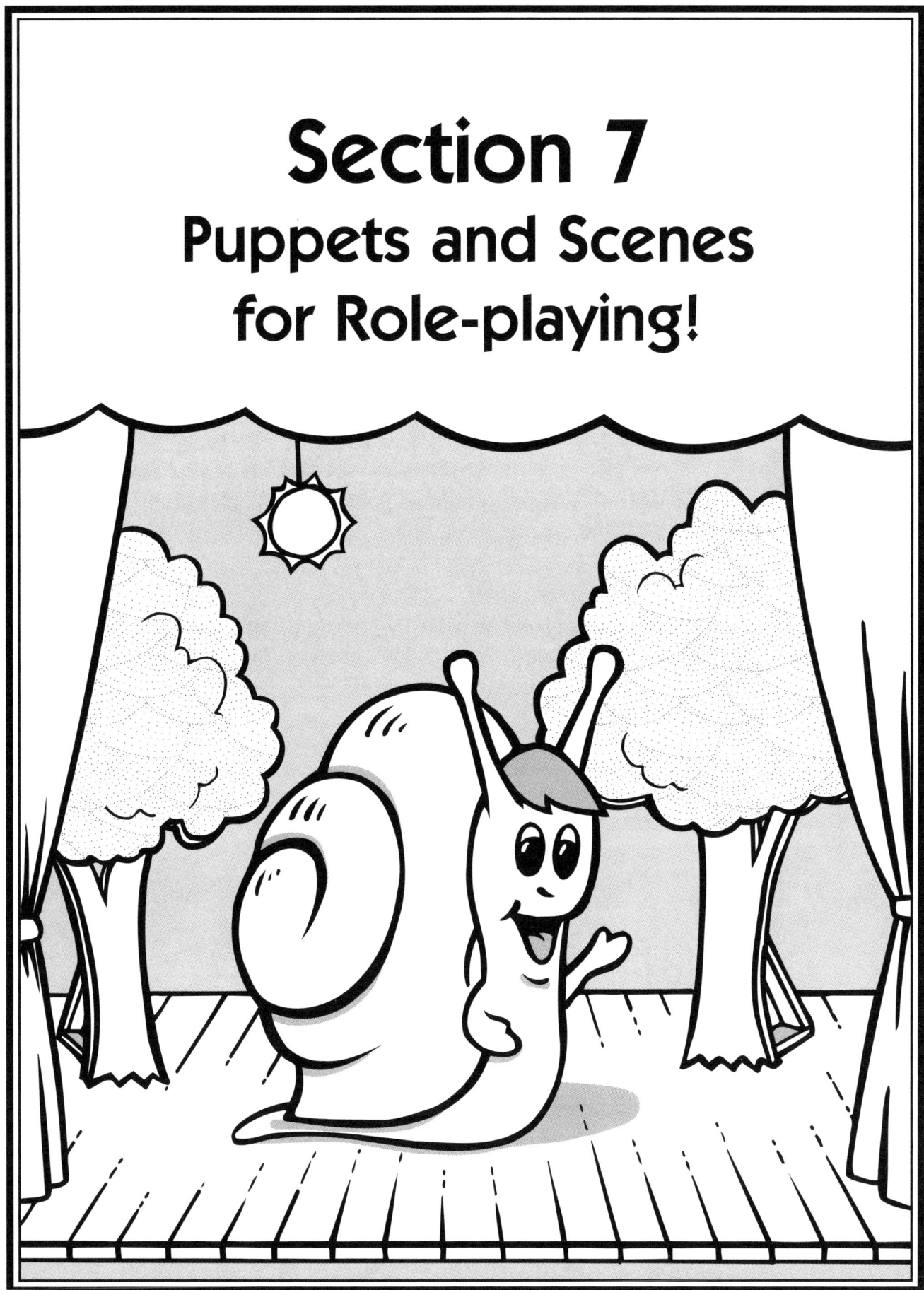

Puppet Instructions

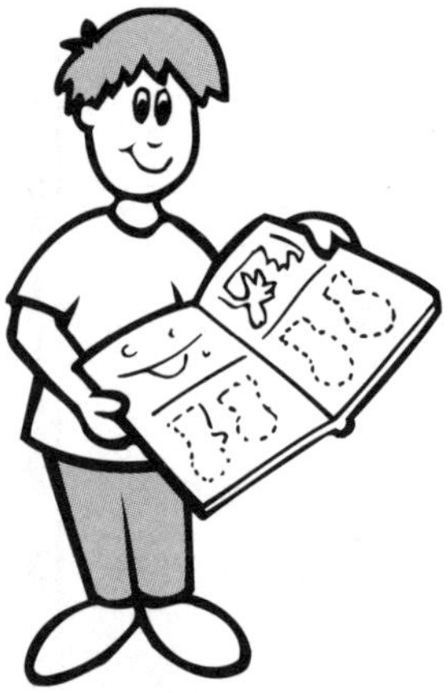

☐ Choose puppet scene desired (i.e. "The Castle"). Photocopy entire page.

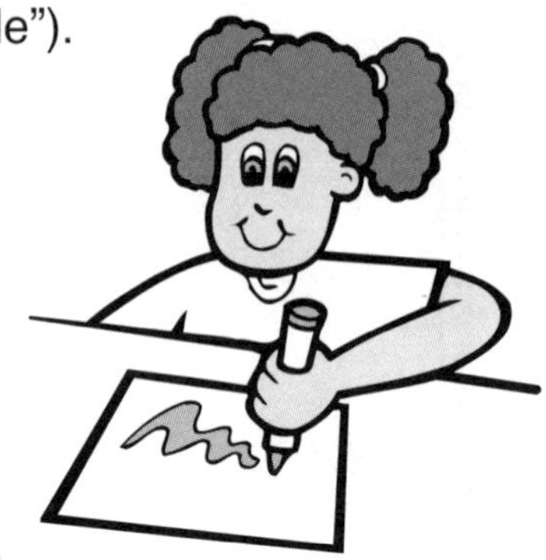

☐ Have child color the scene and the puppets.

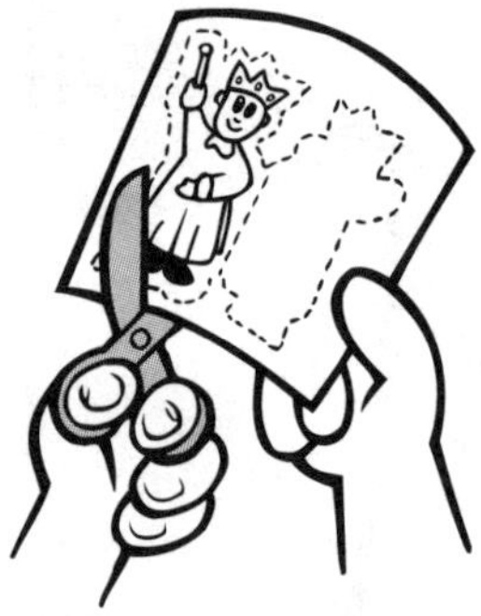

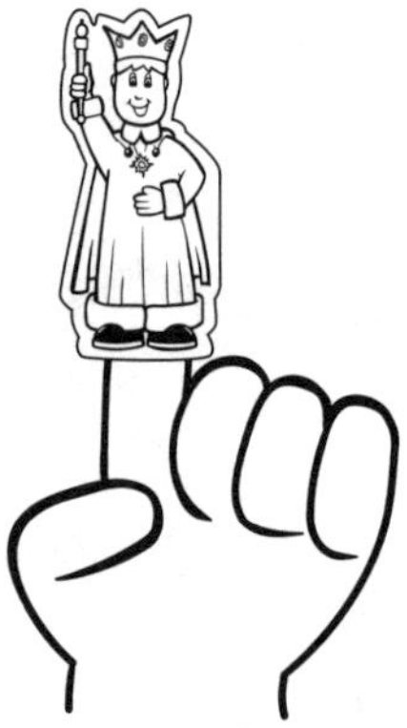

☐ Cut out the puppets. Fold in half. Glue edges together or staple leaving an opening for child's finger.

Option: Glue puppet onto a popsicle stick!

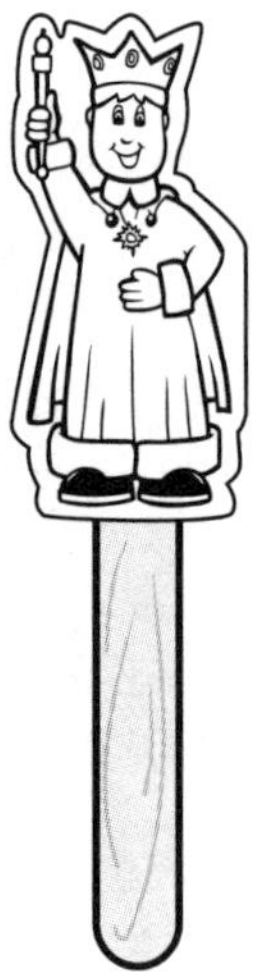

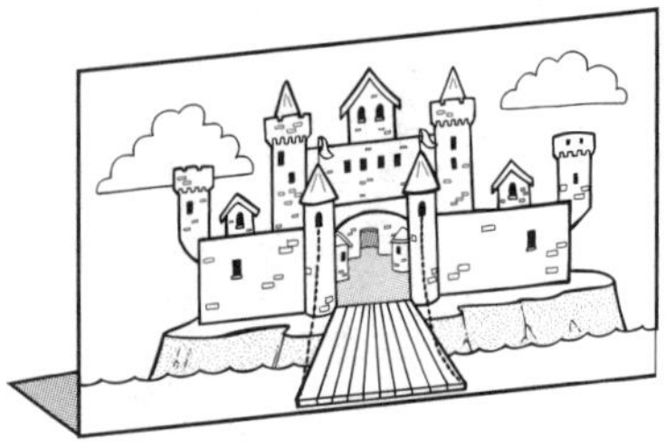

☐ Fold back scene on solid line so that it stands up. It may help to glue scene onto construction paper before folding back. This should make the scene more stable.

☐ Have child pretend to be one of the characters. Encourage the child to talk about the scene using a slow and easy voice.

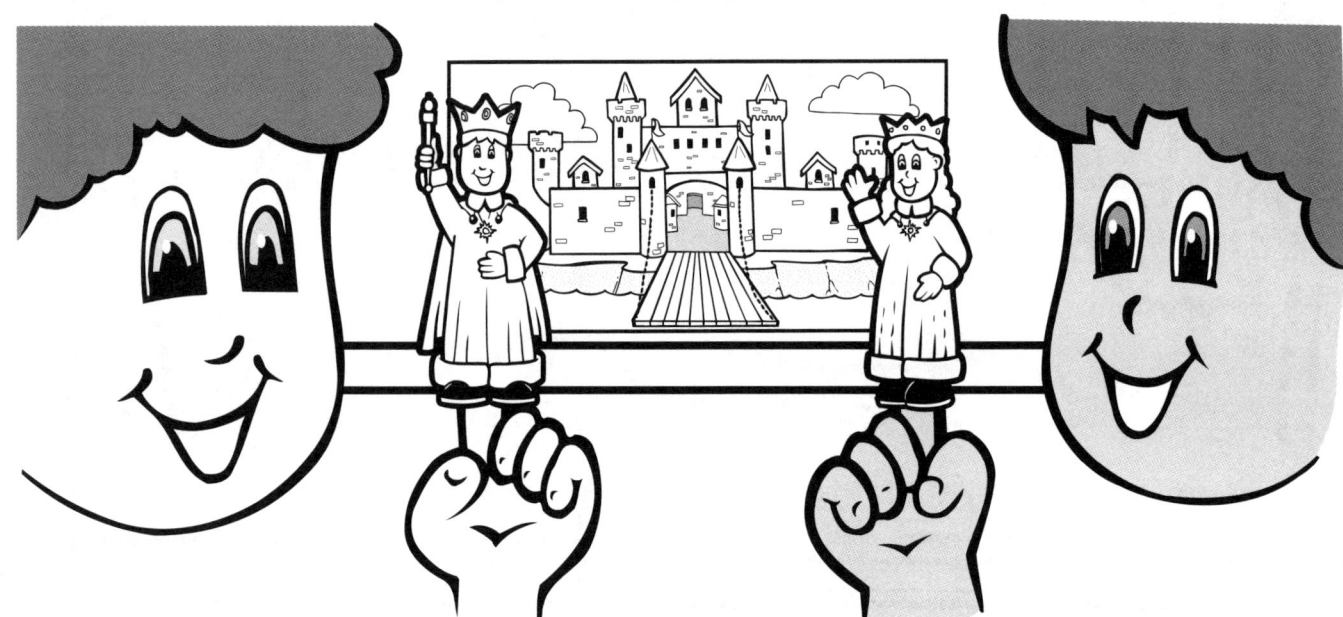

The Castle

Pretend you are a King or Queen. Tell Snooky what it is like to live in a castle. Use your slow and easy voice.

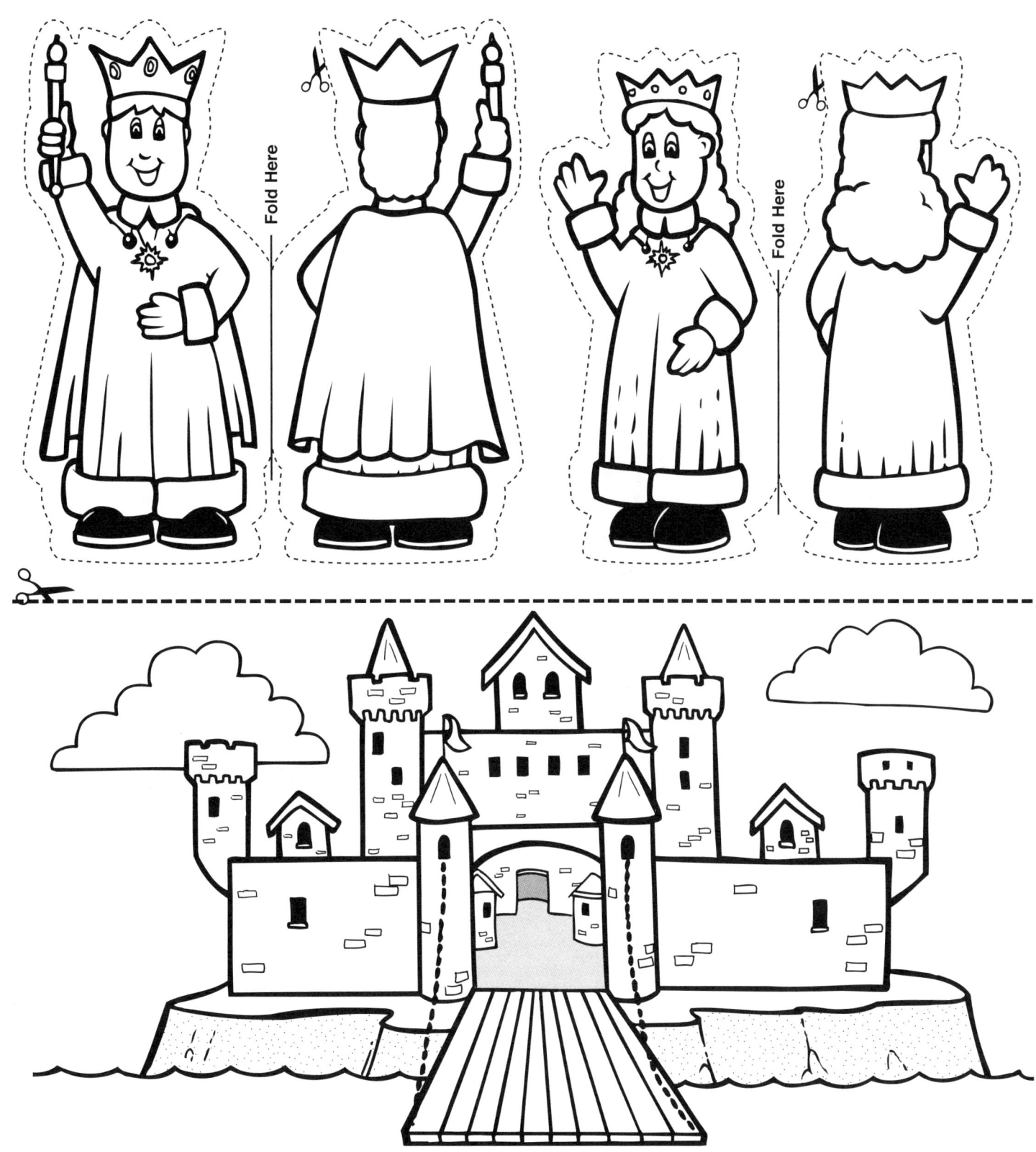

Fantasy Garden

Pretend you are a unicorn or a fairy. Tell Snooky where you live and all about your magical powers. Use your slow and easy voice.

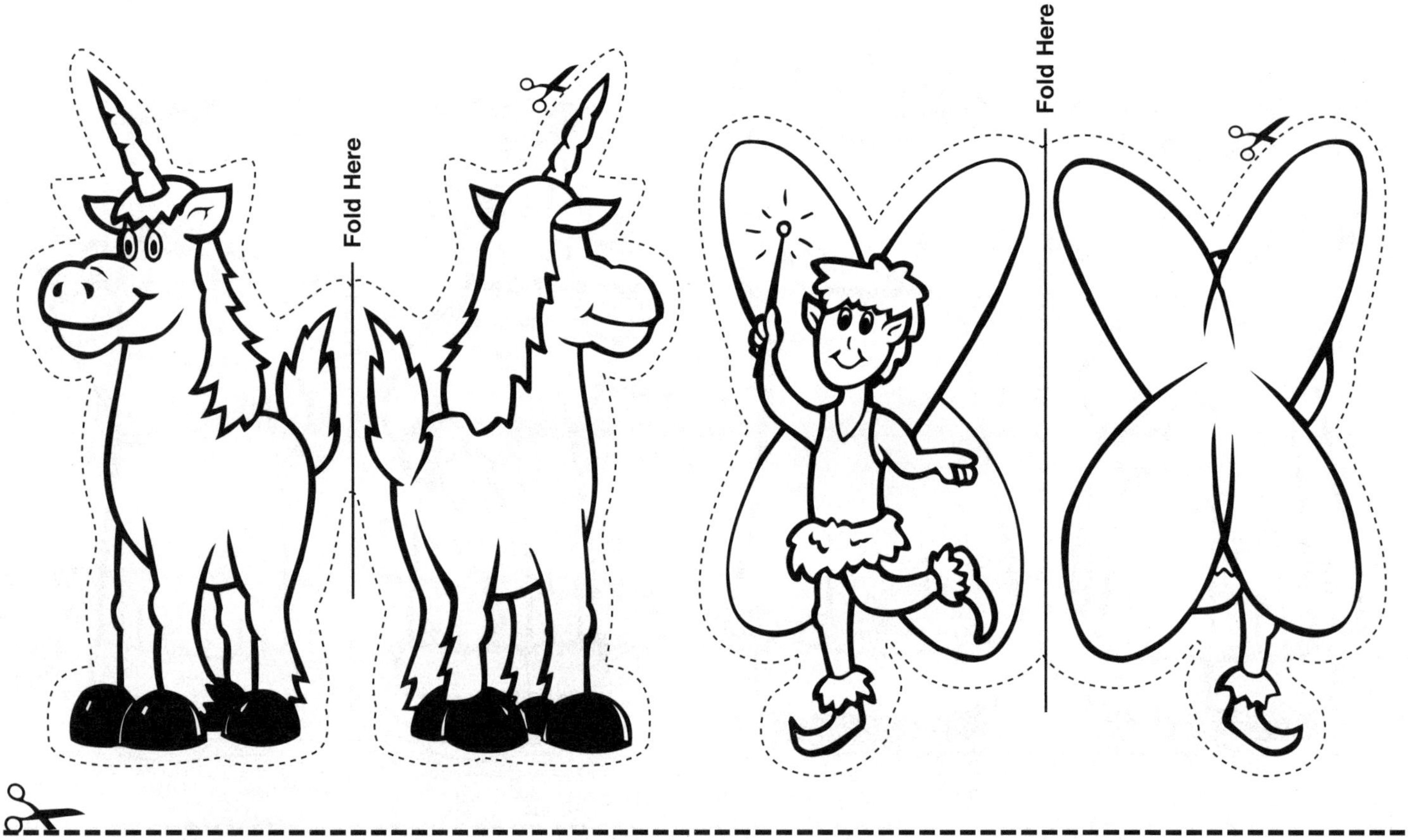

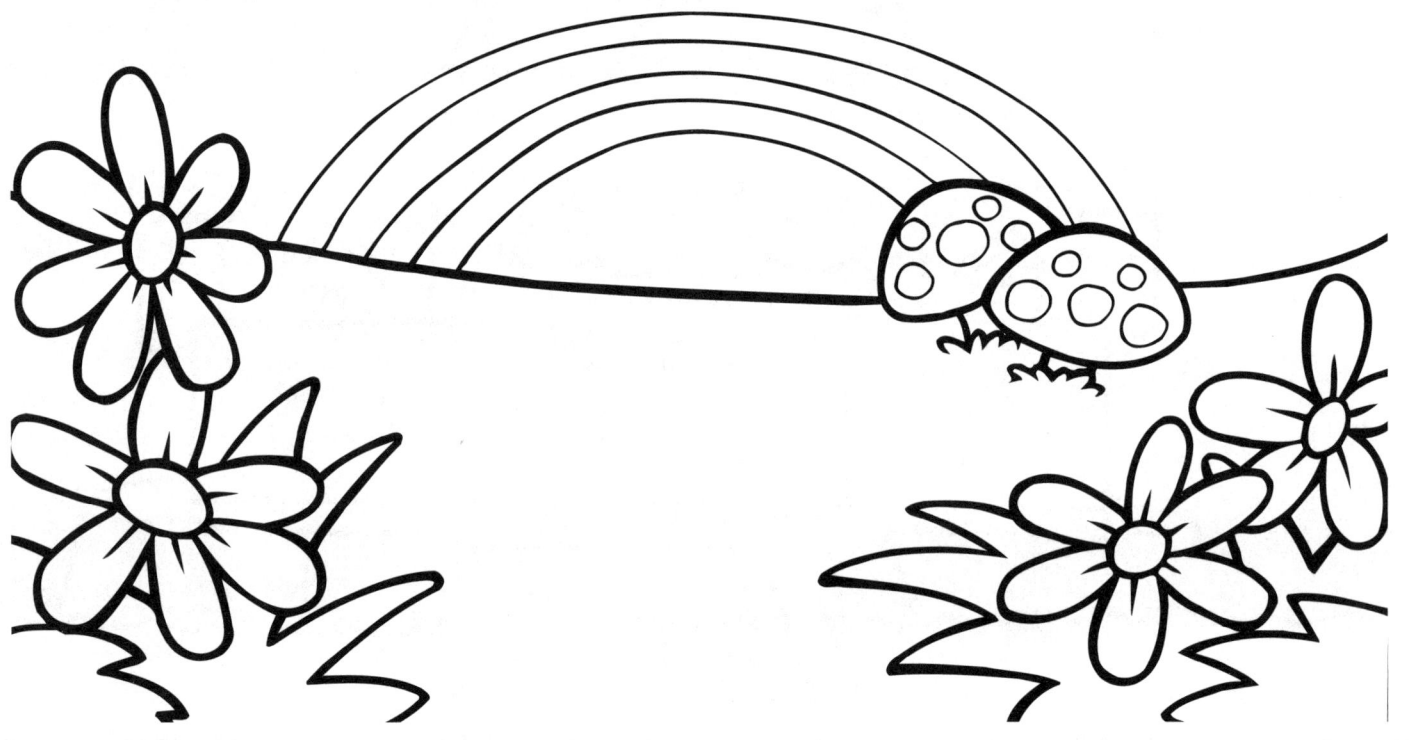

Fold Back Here   Fold Back Here

Jungle Scene

Pretend you are a monkey or a lion. Tell Snooky what it is like to live in the jungle. Use your slow and easy voice.

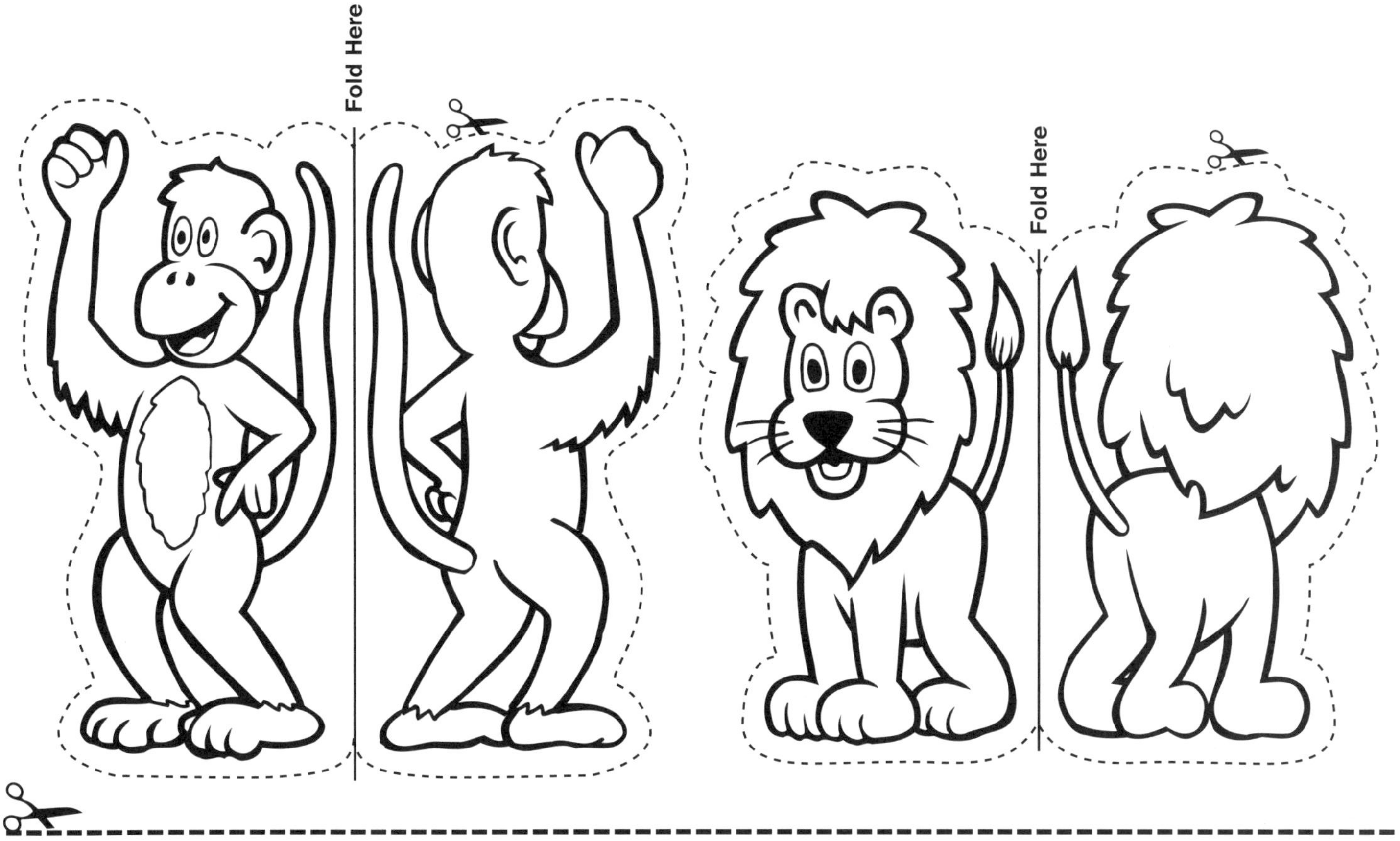

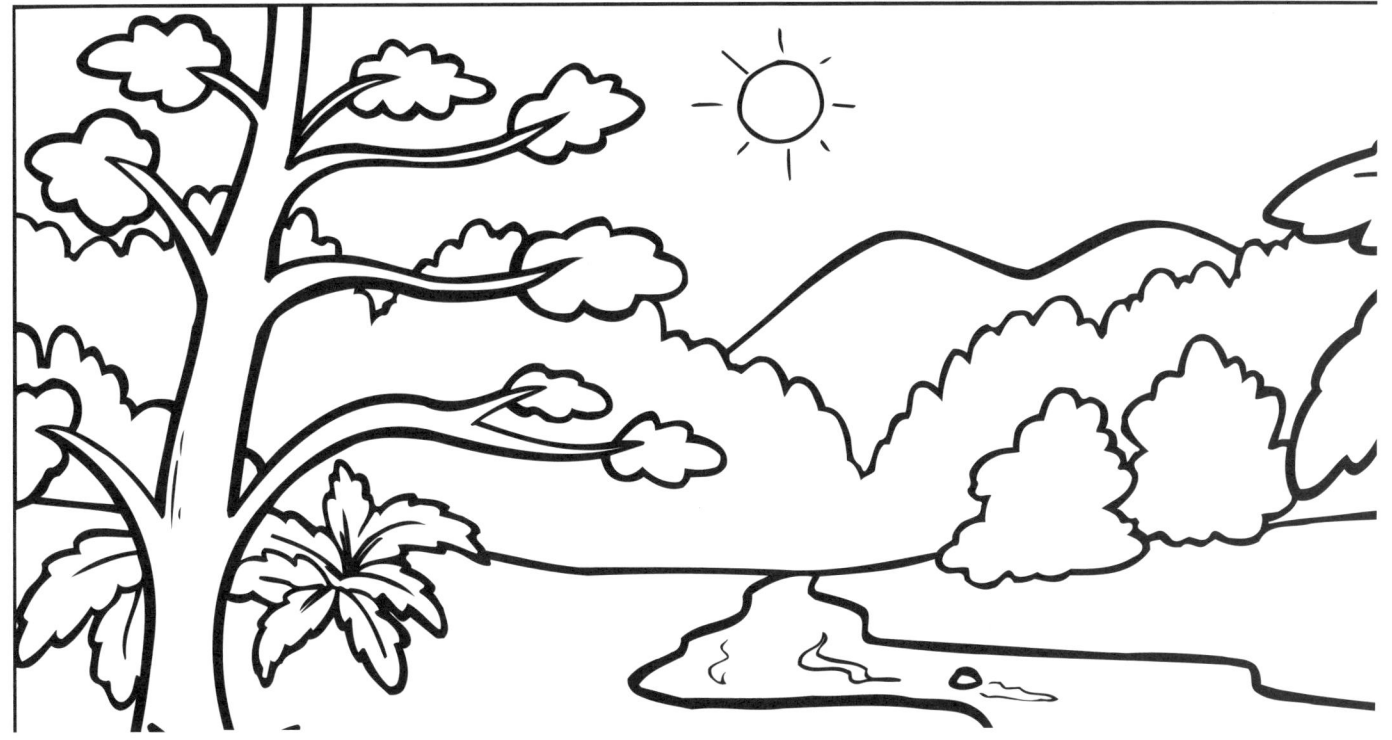

Fold Back Here   Fold Back Here

Under the Sea

Pretend you are a whale or a starfish. Tell Snooky what it is like to live under the sea. Who are your friends? Use your slow and easy voice.

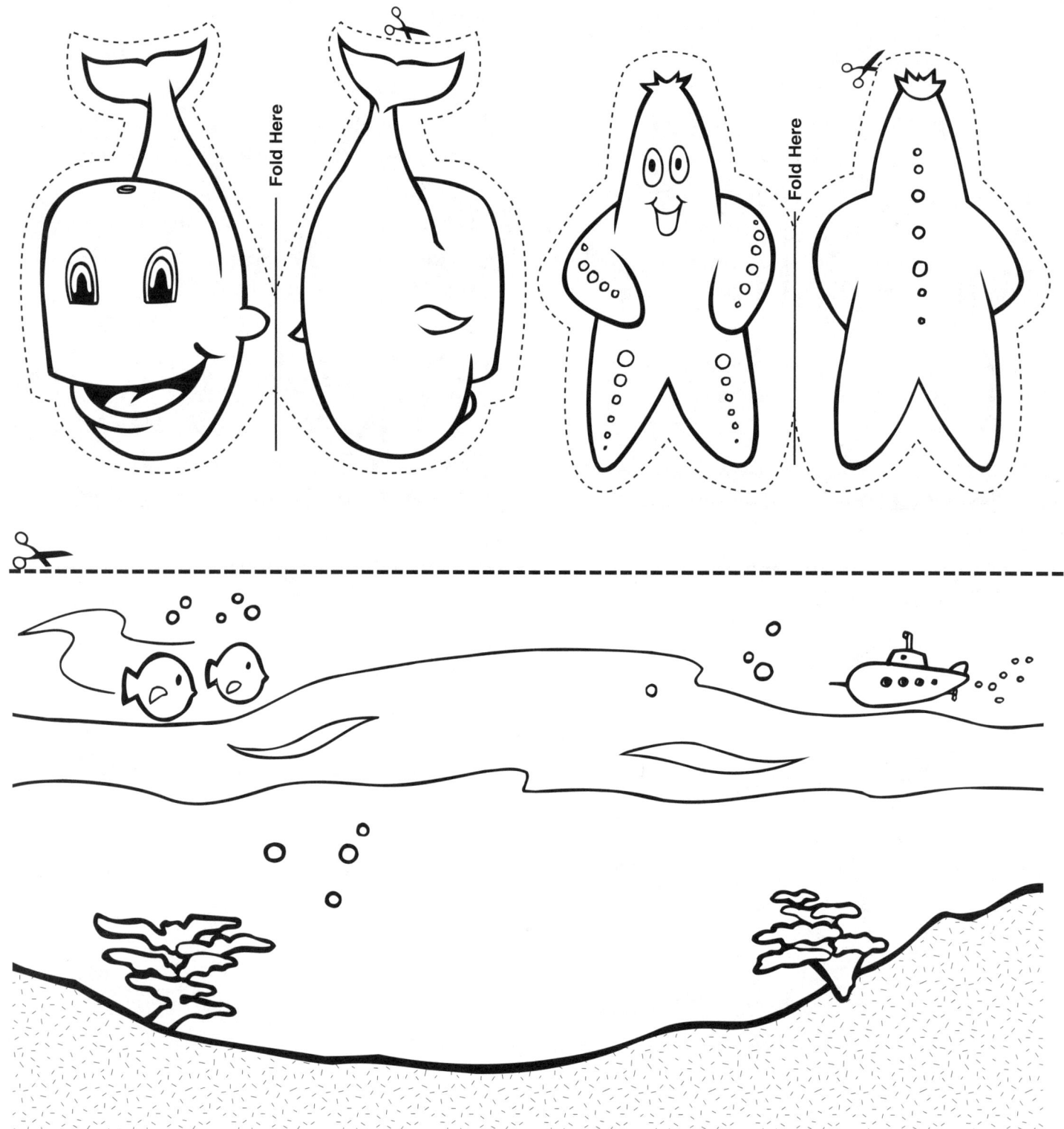

Alien Planet

Tell Snooky what it is like to live on another planet and what you like about Earth. Use your slow and easy voice.

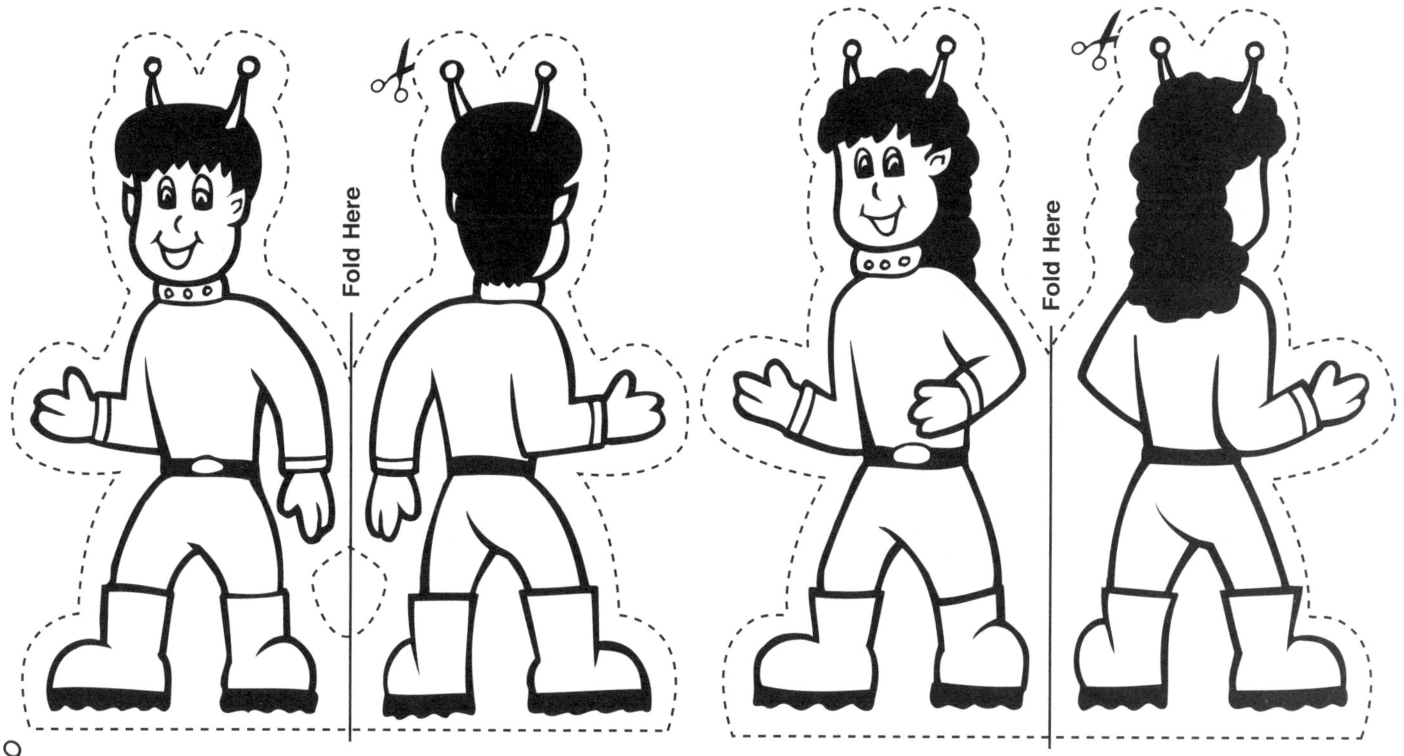

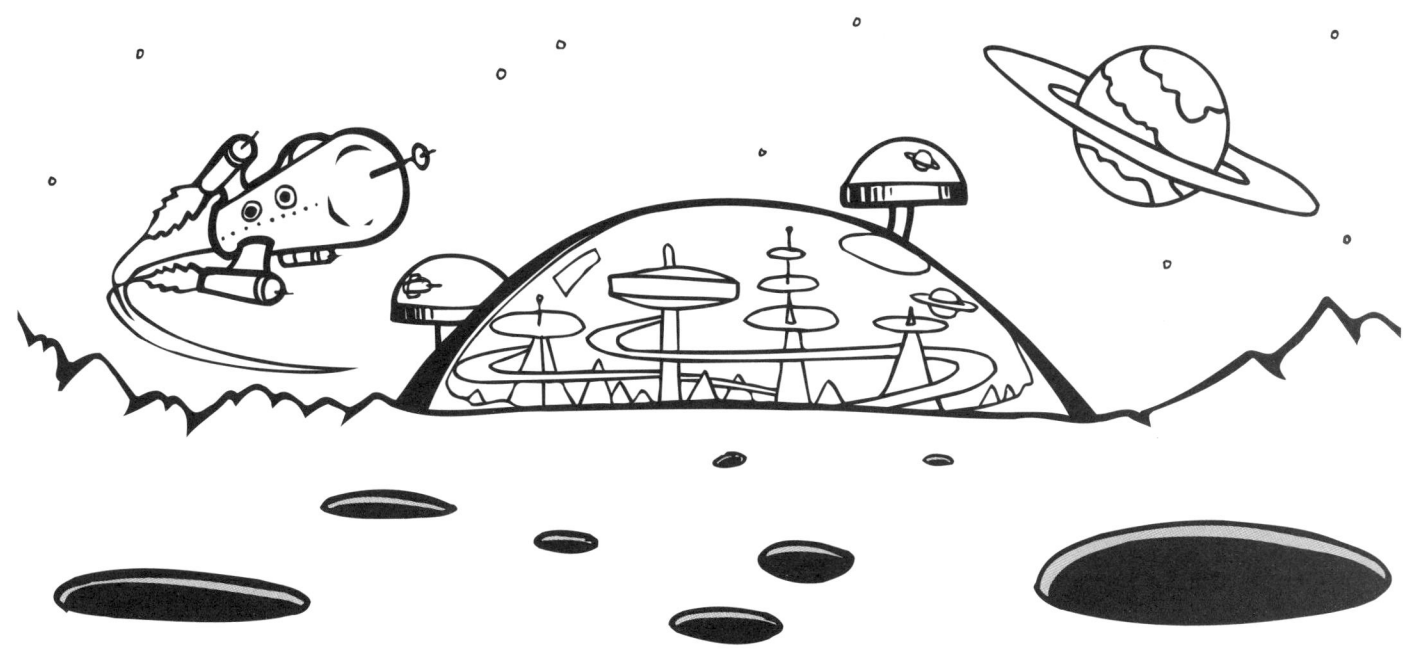

The Fire Station

Pretend you are a firefighter. Tell Snooky what your job is like. Describe the fire engine. Use your slow and easy voice.

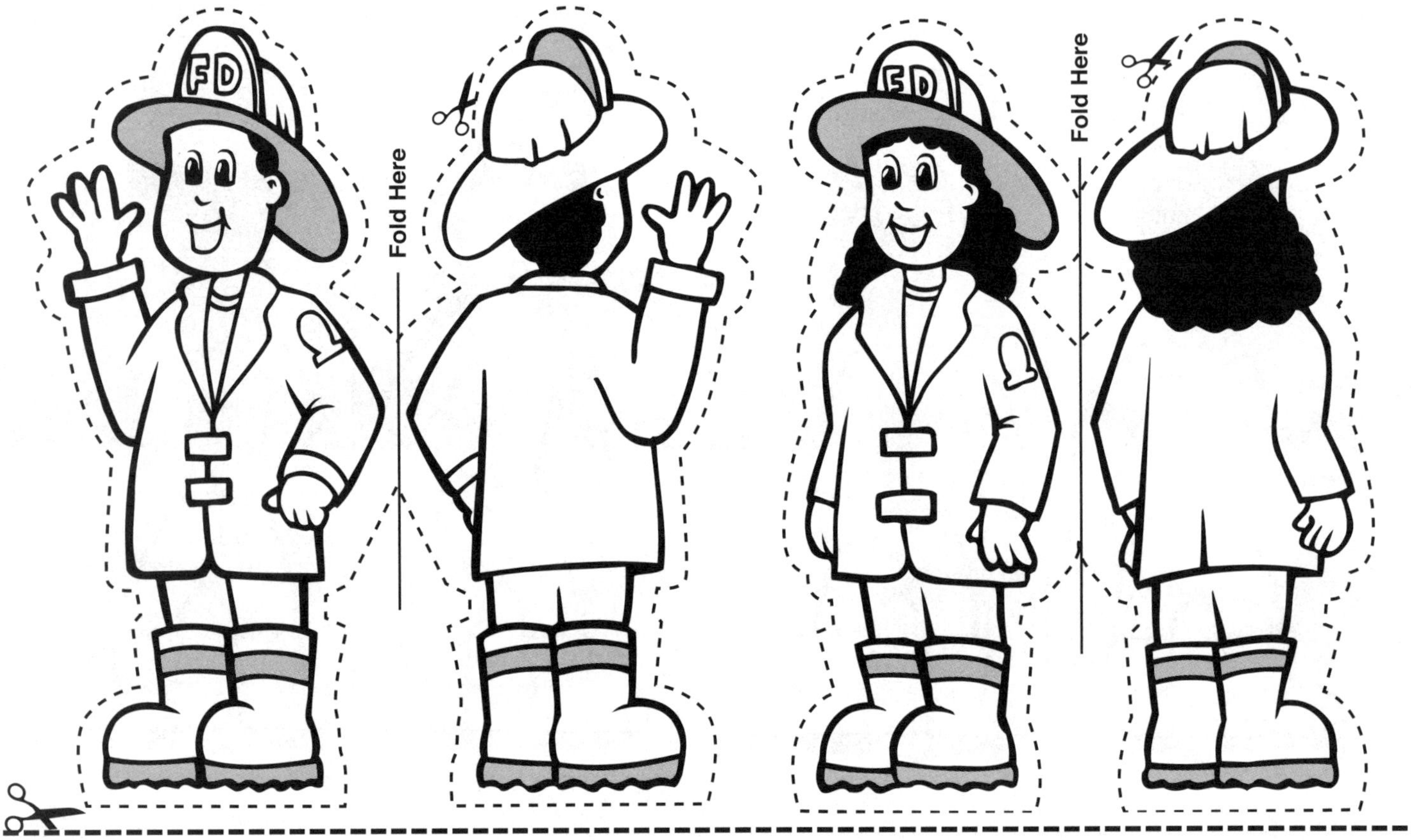

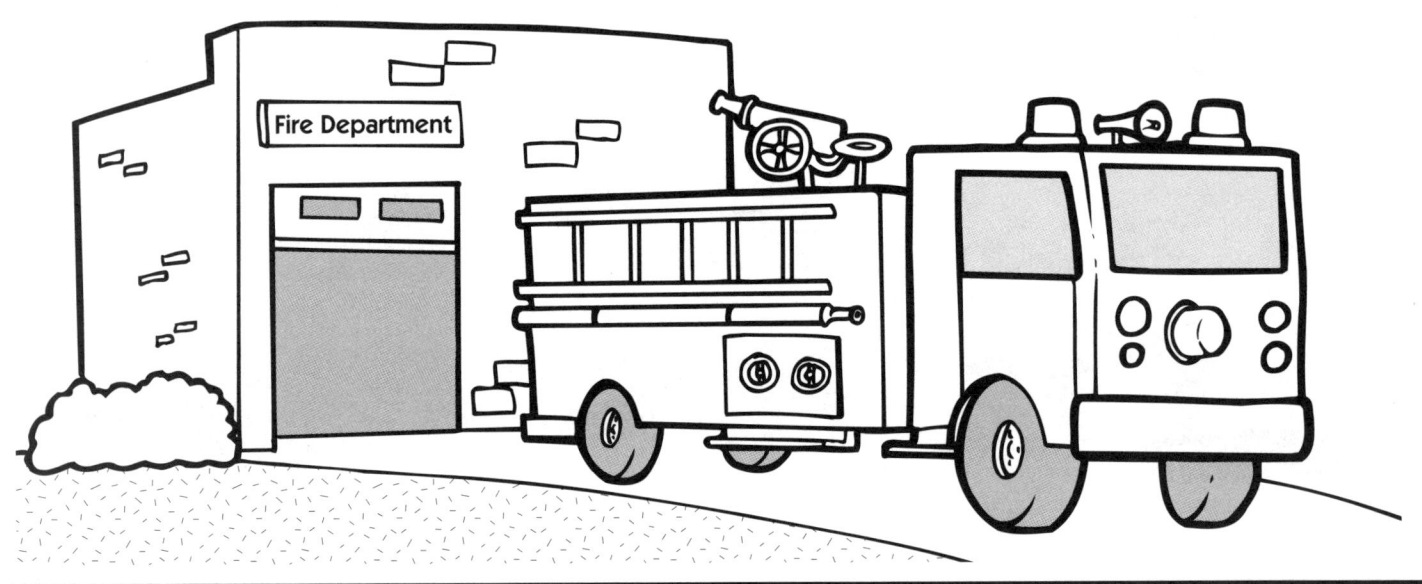

Fold Back Here   Fold Back Here

At the Circus

Pretend you are a clown or a trapeze person in the circus. What is it like to swing so high in the air? If you are a clown, how do you make people laugh? Use your slow and easy voice.

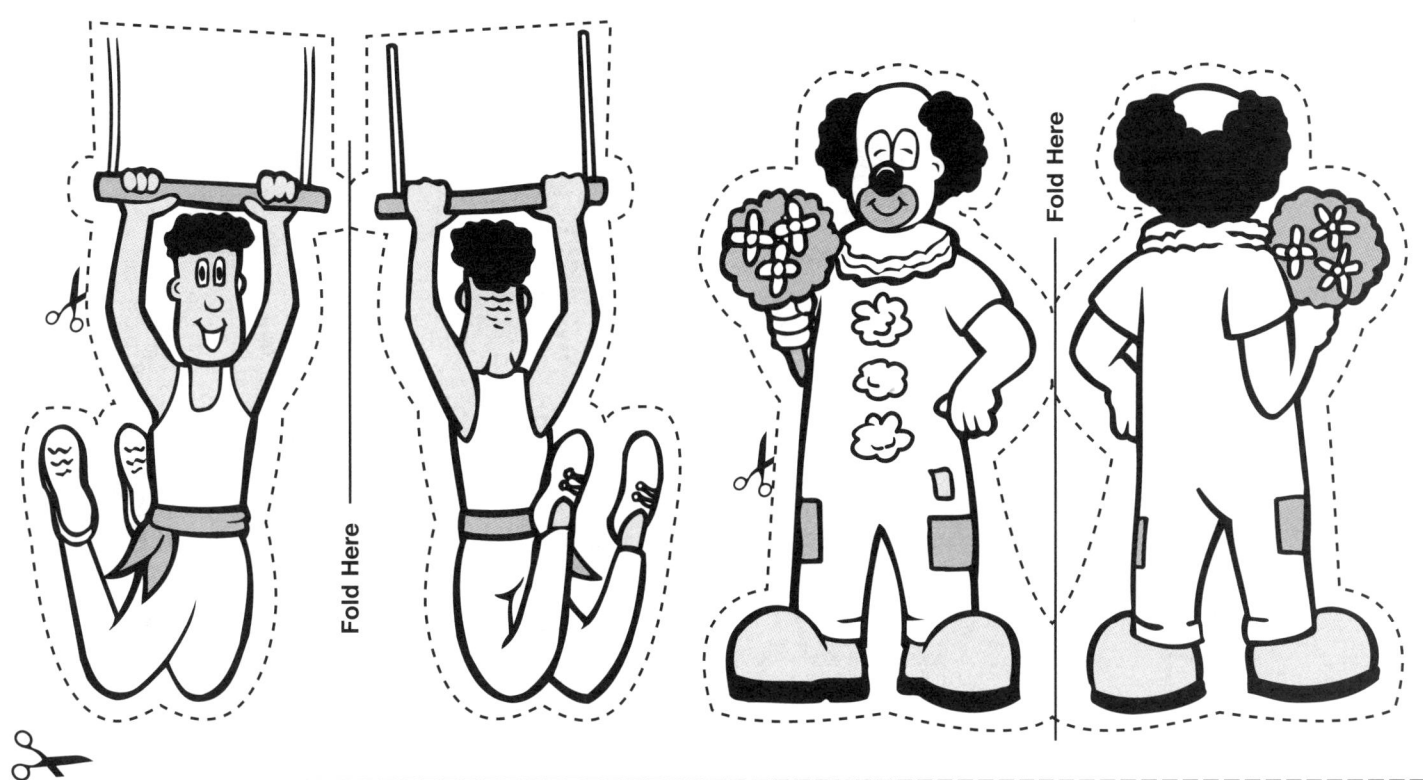

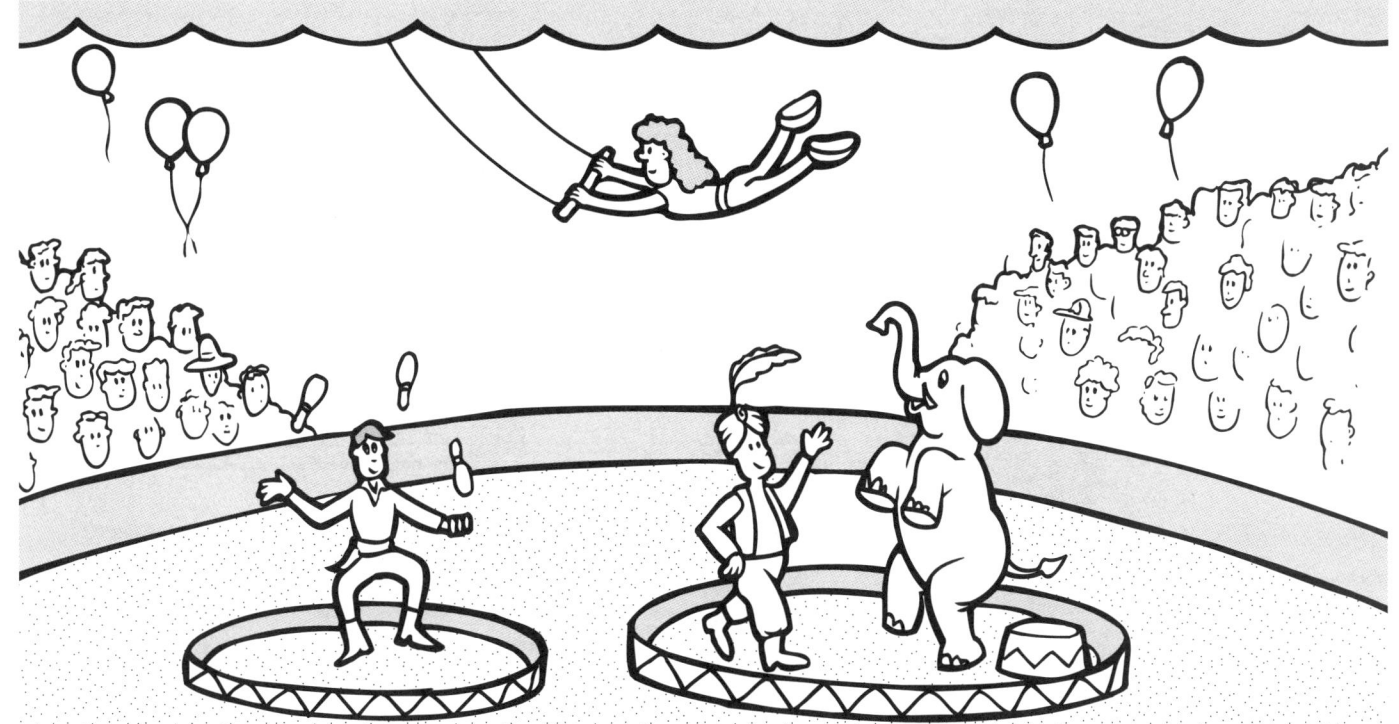

Fold Back Here · Fold Back Here

Police Officer

Pretend you are a police officer. Tell Snooky all about your job and your patrol car. Use your slow and easy voice.

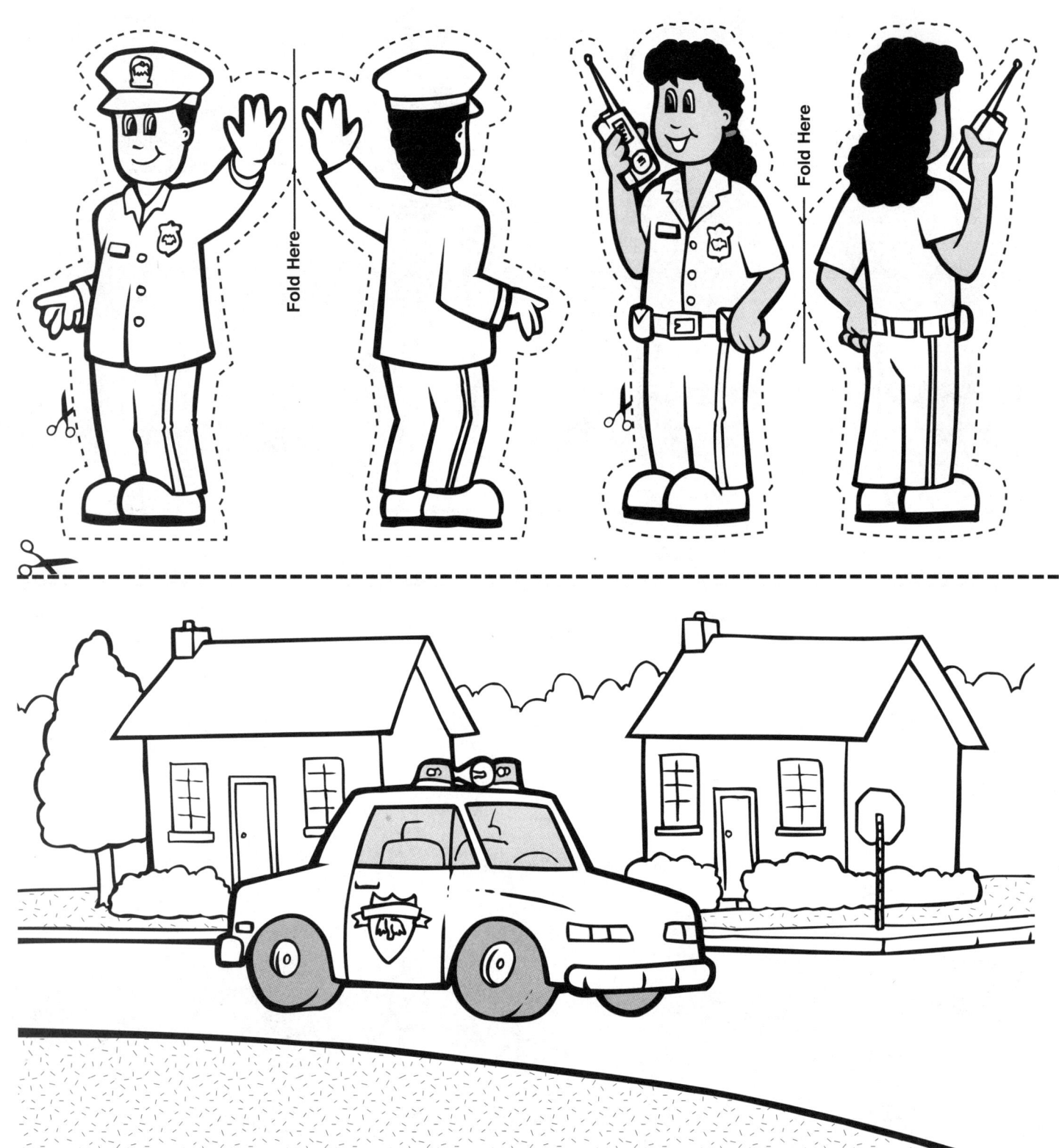

On the Farm

Pretend you are a farmer. Tell Snooky all about the farm and your favorite animal. Use your slow and easy voice.

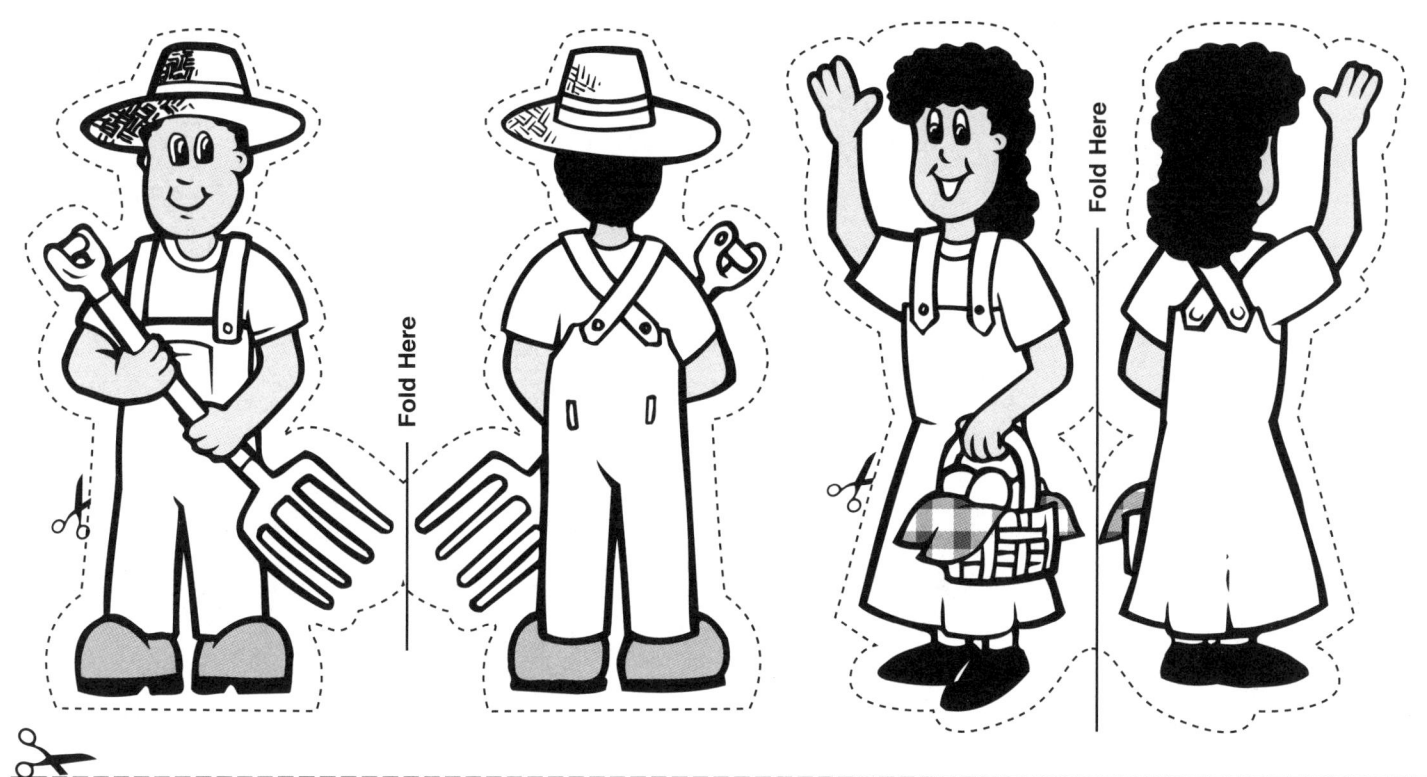

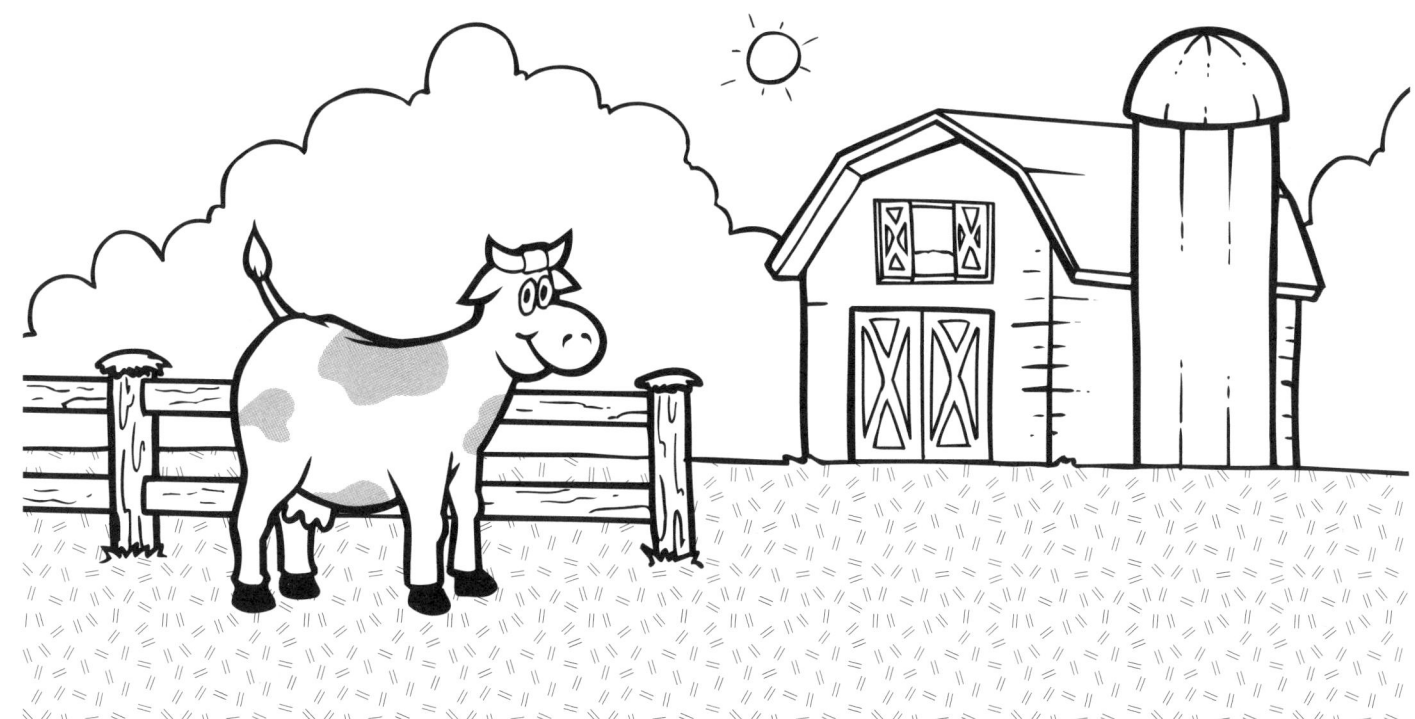

Fold Back Here	Fold Back Here

The North Pole

Pretend you are Santa Claus or one of his reindeer. Tell Snooky about Christmas. If you are a reindeer, tell Snooky what it is like to fly. Use your slow and easy voice.

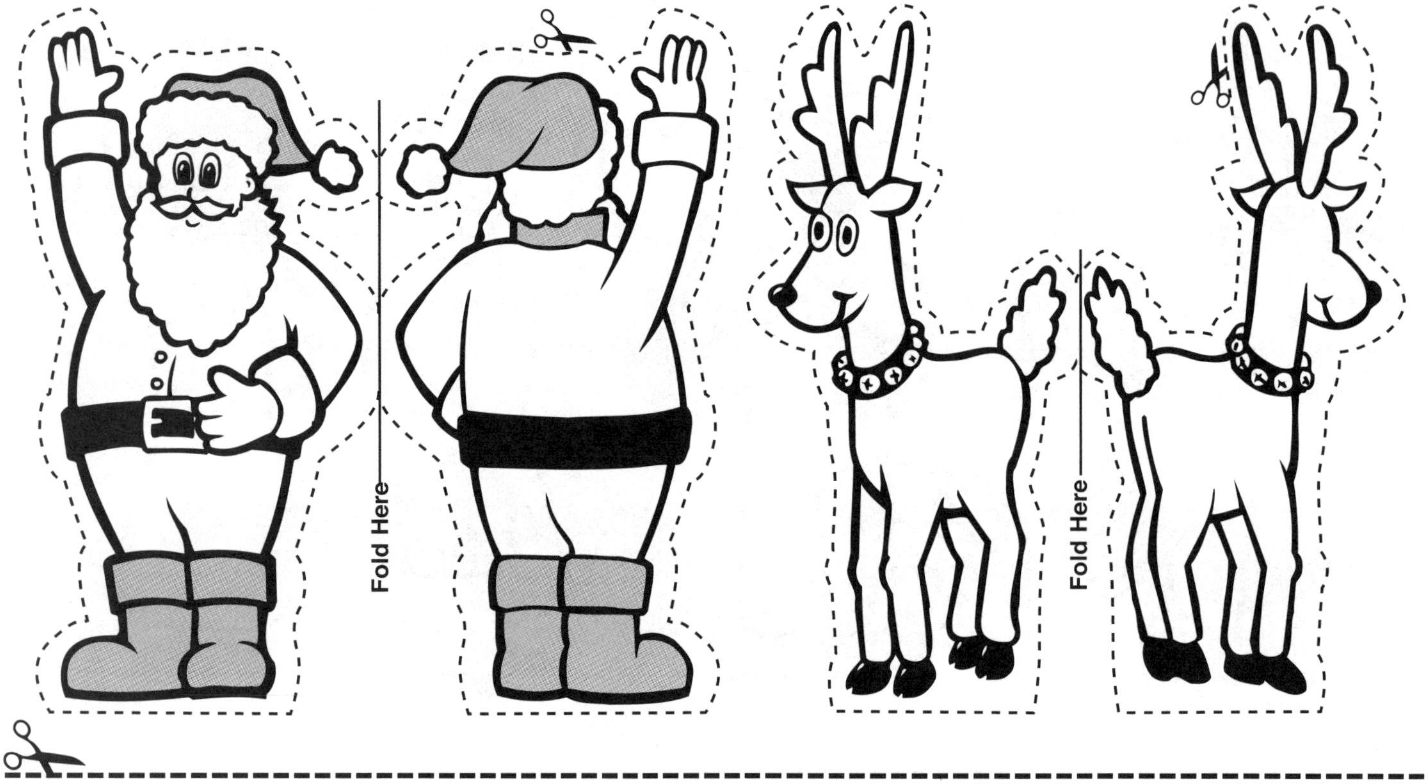

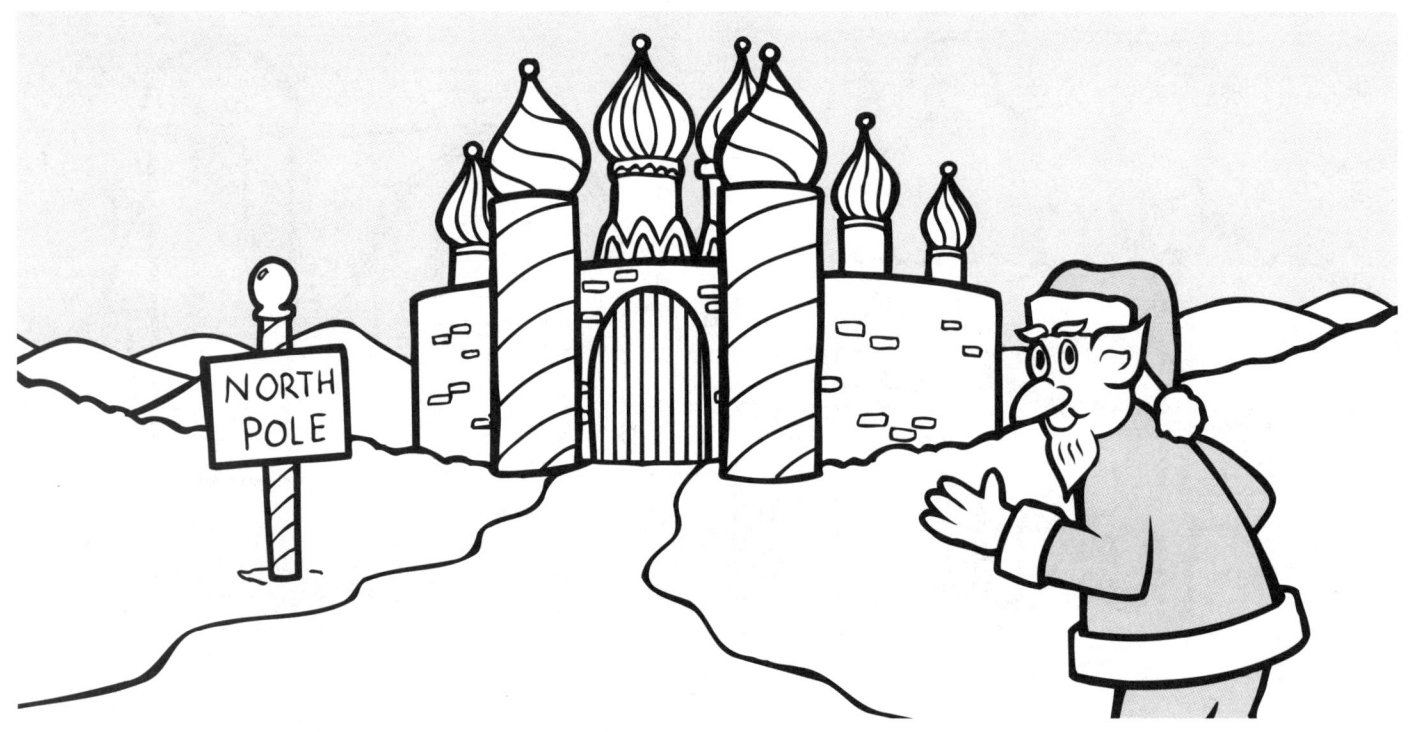

Fold Back Here   Fold Back Here

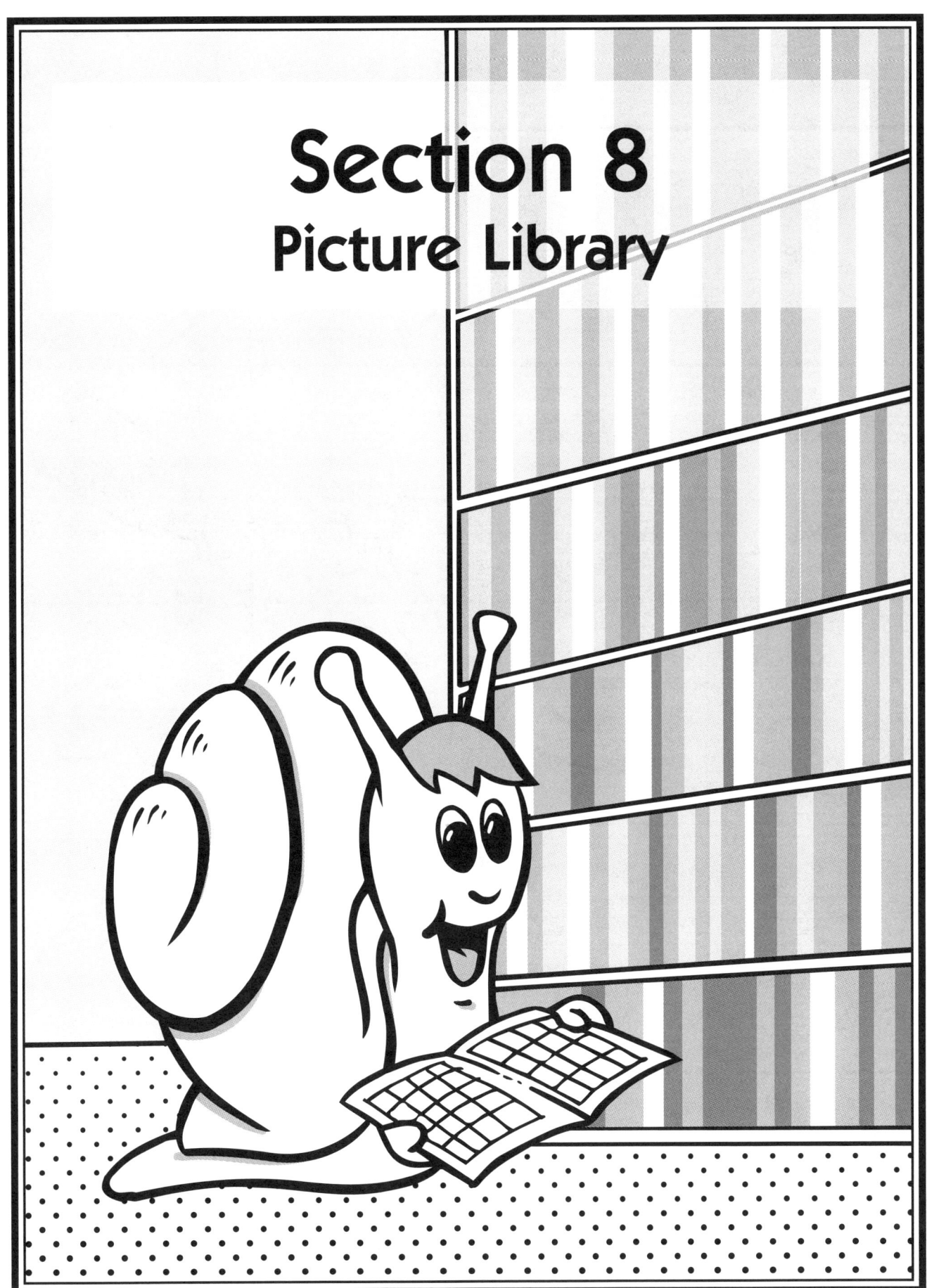

Beach

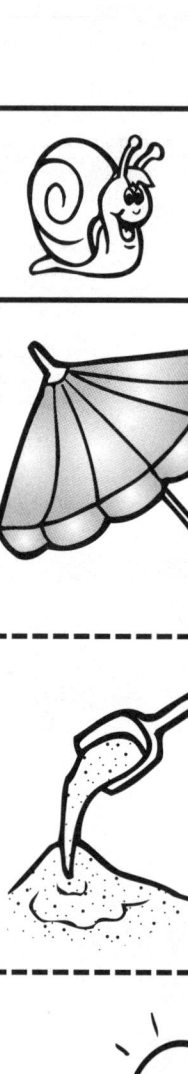
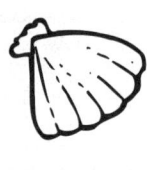
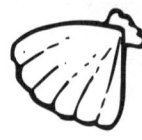
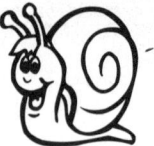
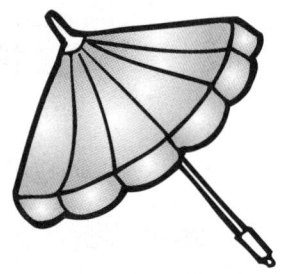
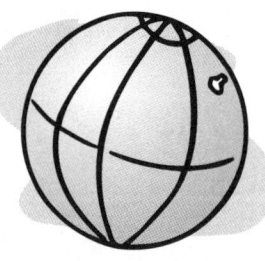
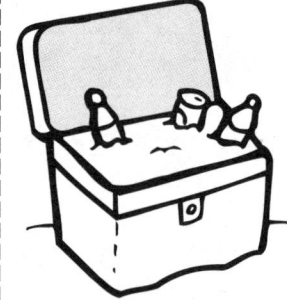
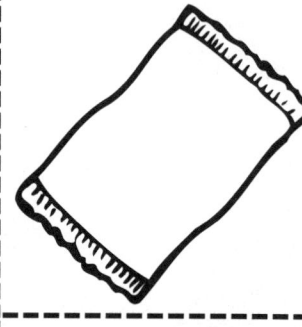
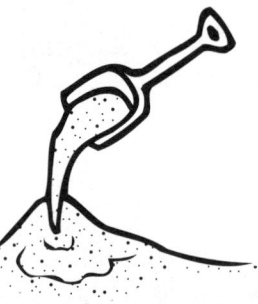
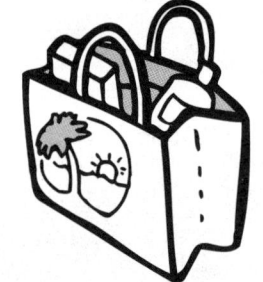
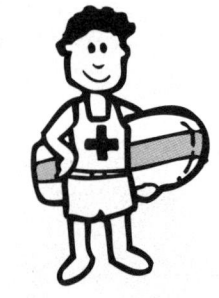
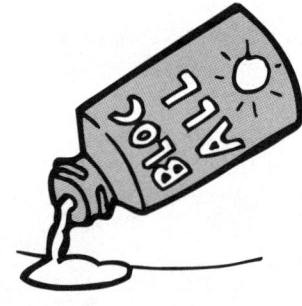

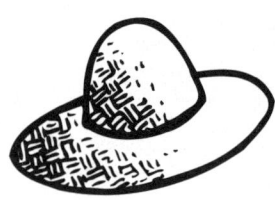
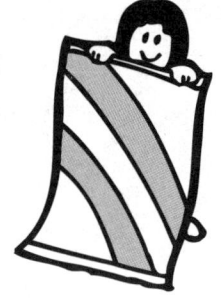
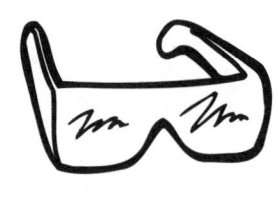

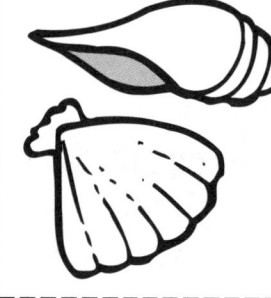
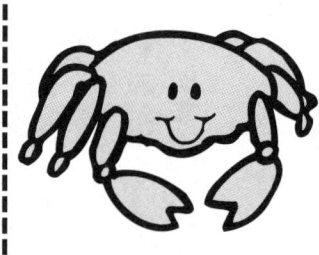
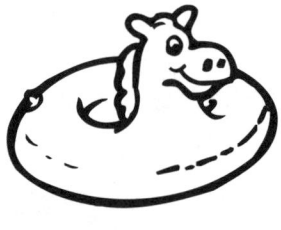
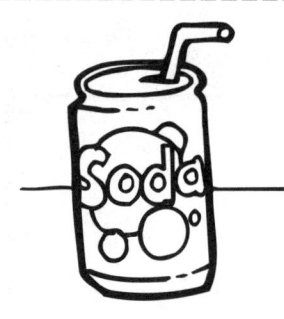
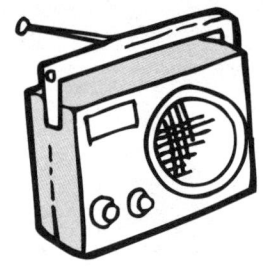
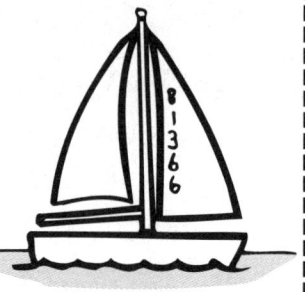
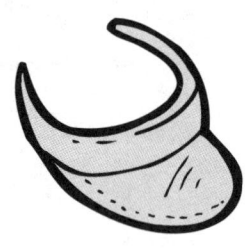

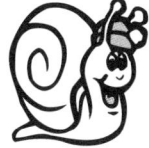 # Bedroom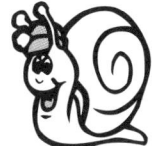

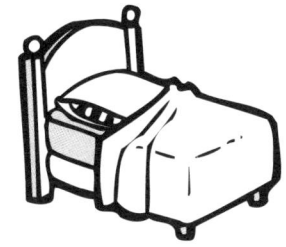 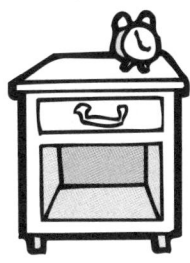  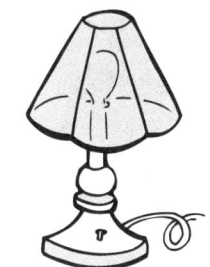

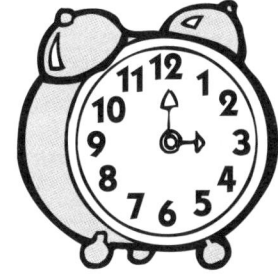 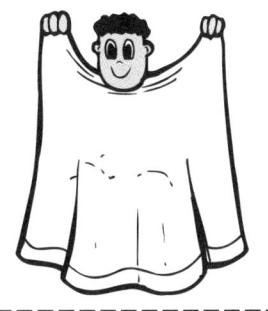 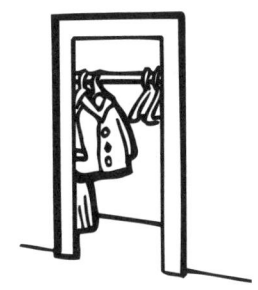 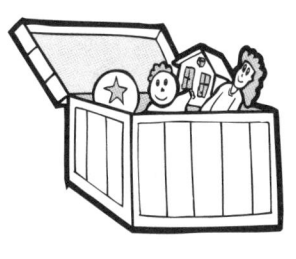

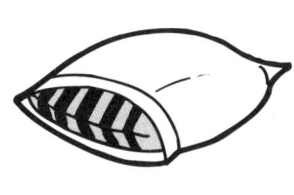 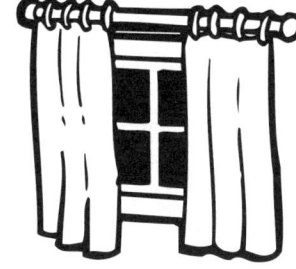 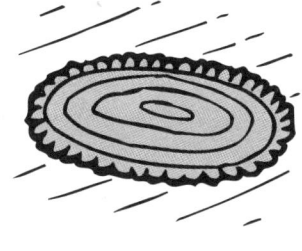 

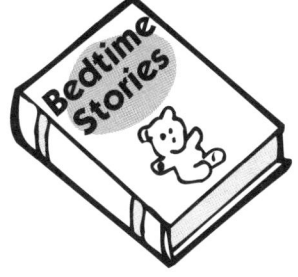 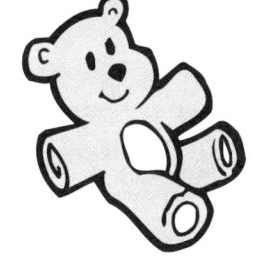 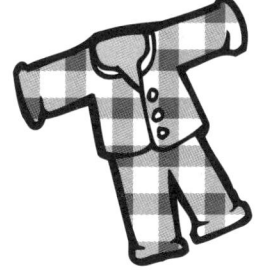 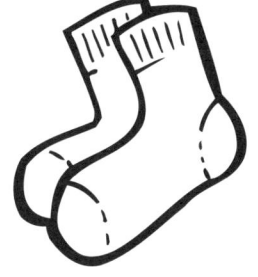

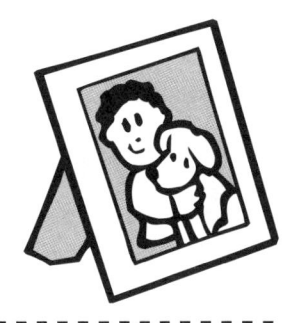 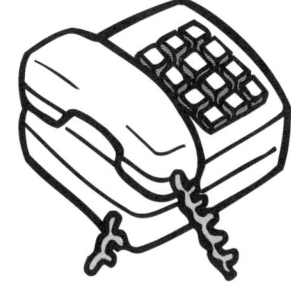 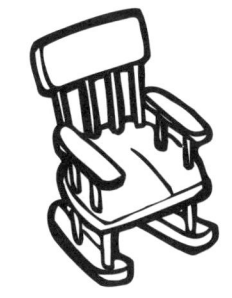 

Christmas/Easter

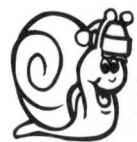 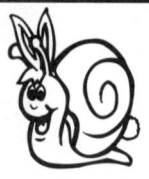

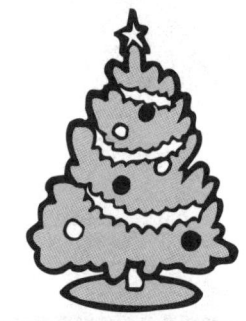 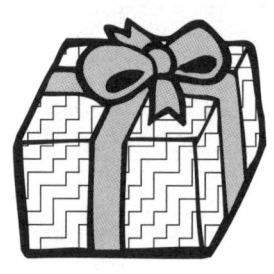  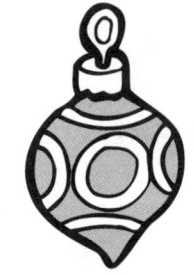

  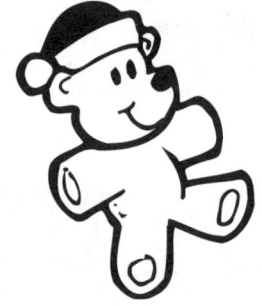 

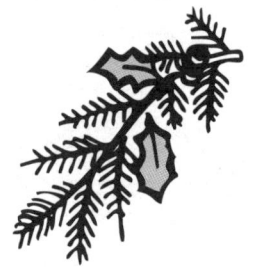 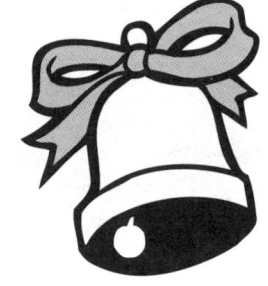  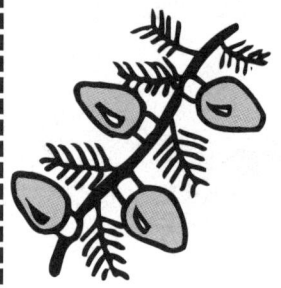

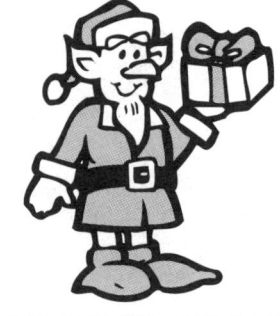 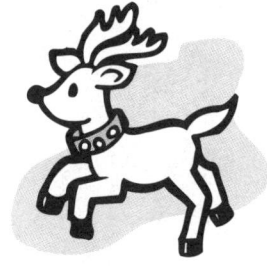 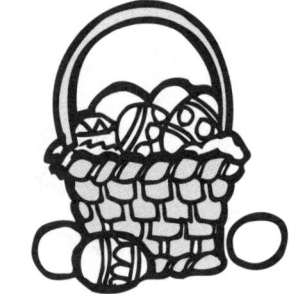 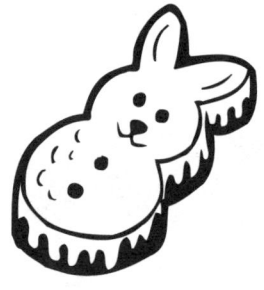

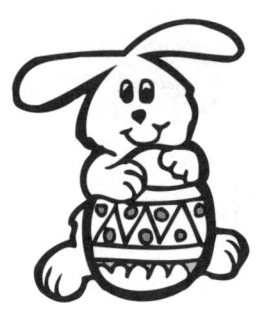 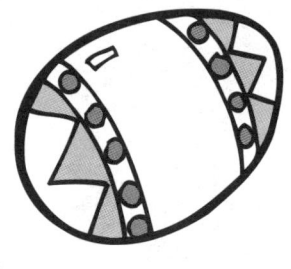 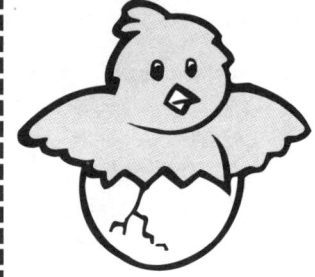 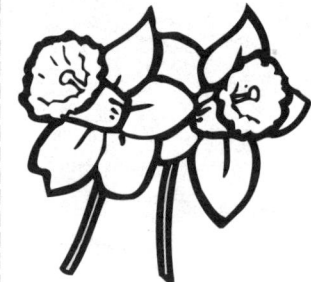

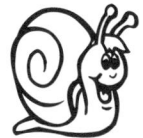 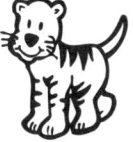 # Circus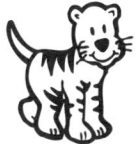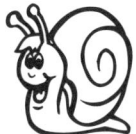

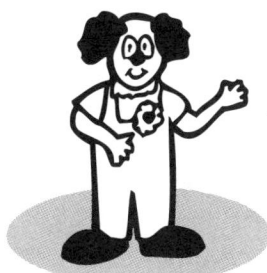 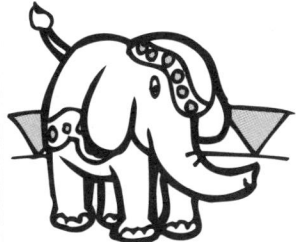 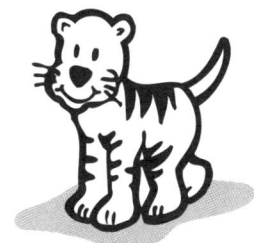 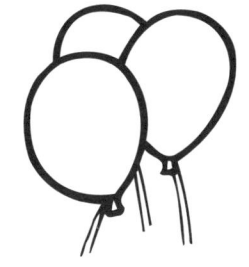

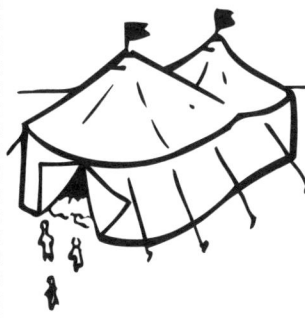 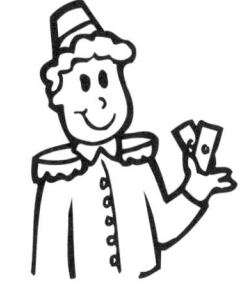 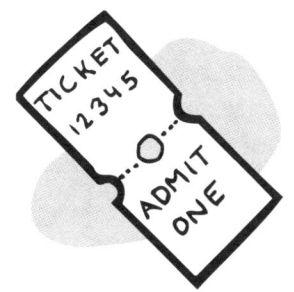 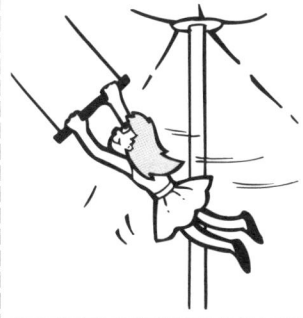

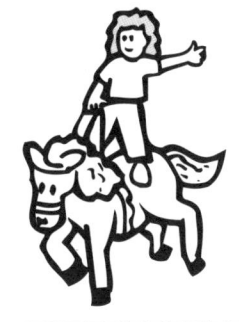 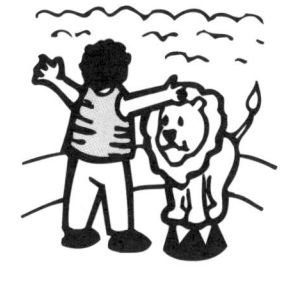 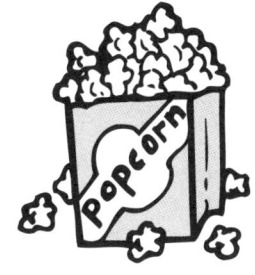 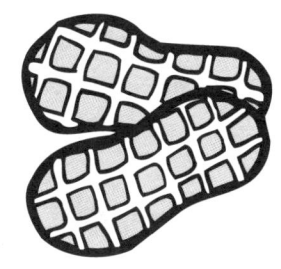

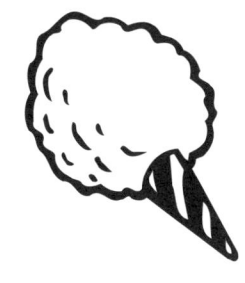 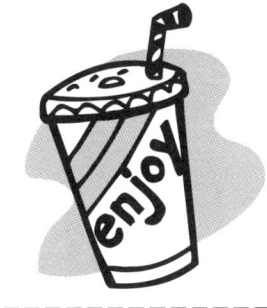 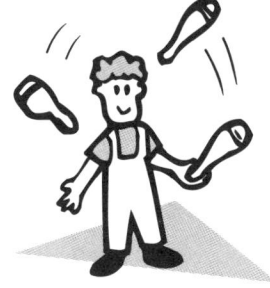 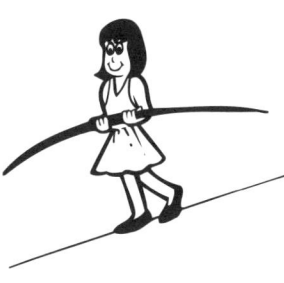

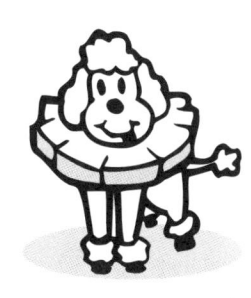 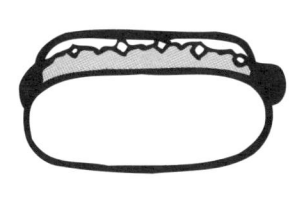 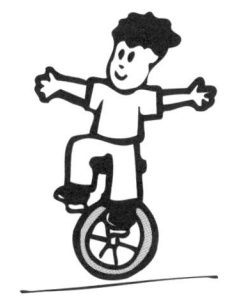 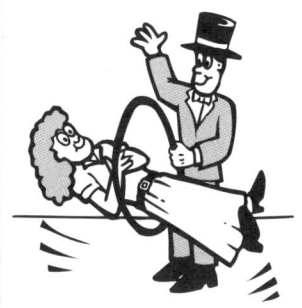

Clothing

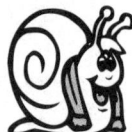 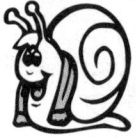

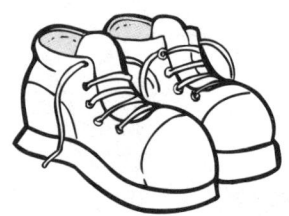 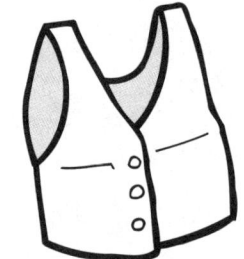 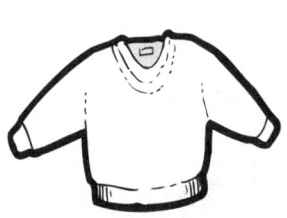 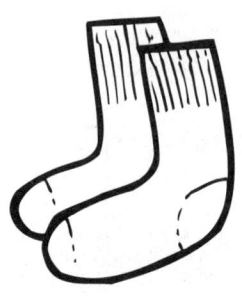

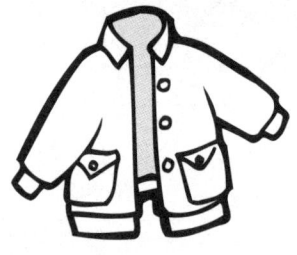 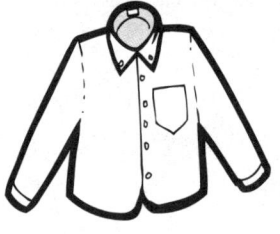 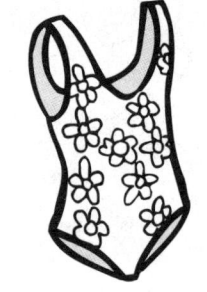 

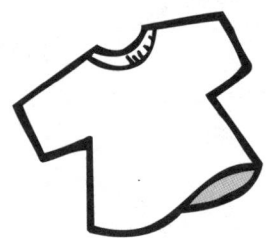 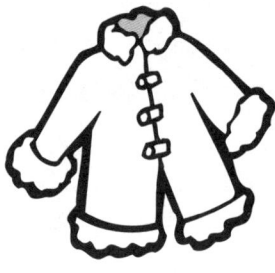 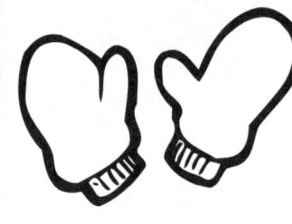 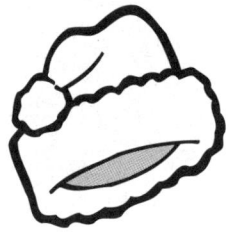

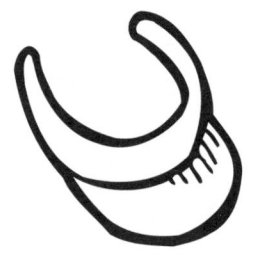 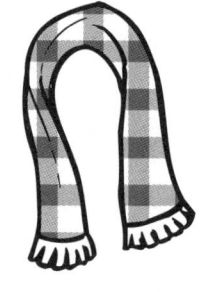 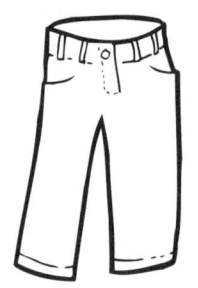 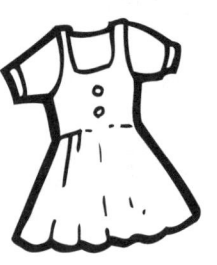

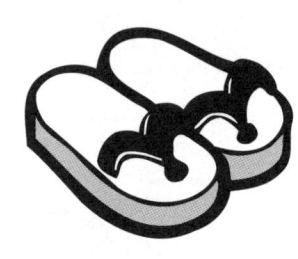 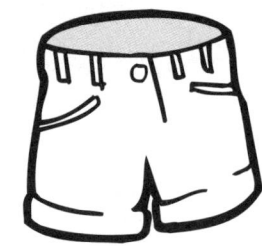 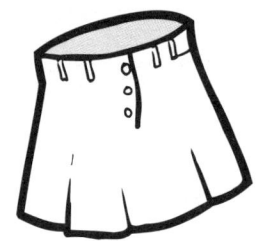 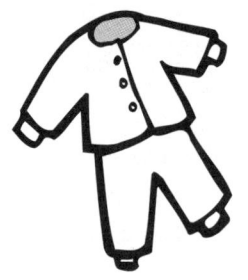

Family & Friends

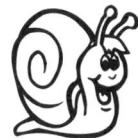
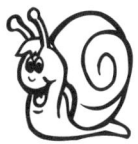
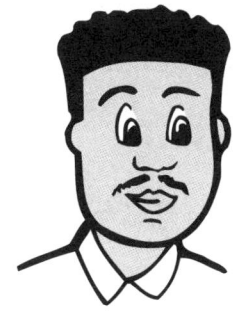
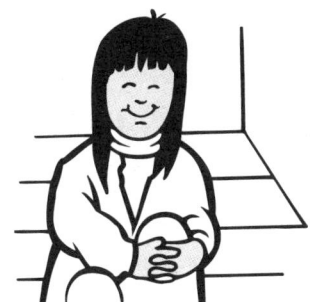
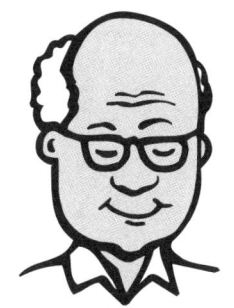
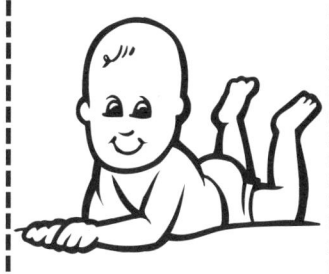
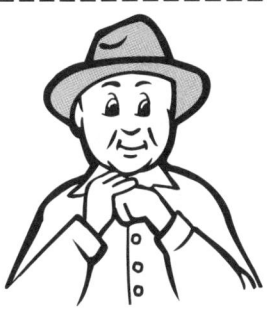
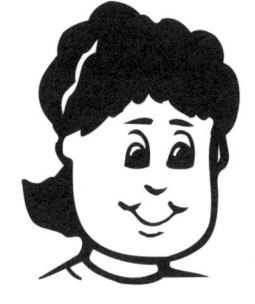
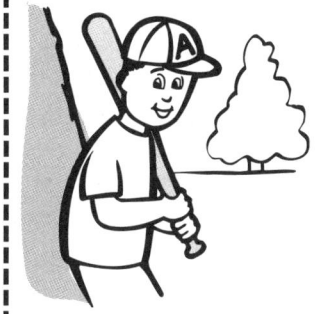
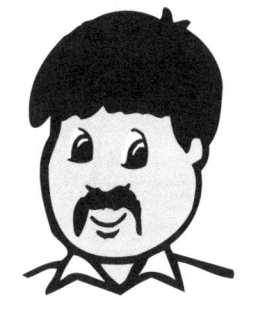
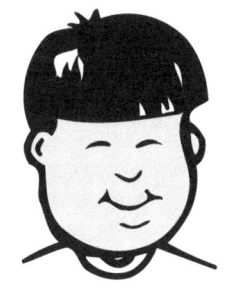
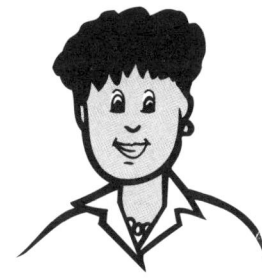
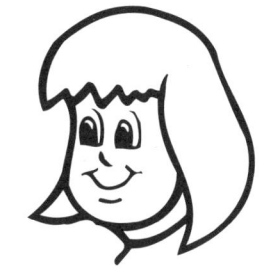
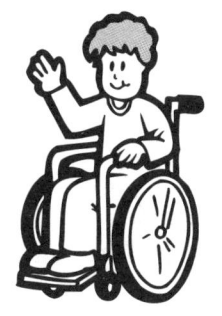
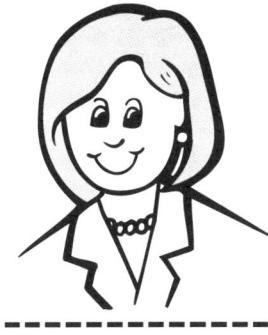
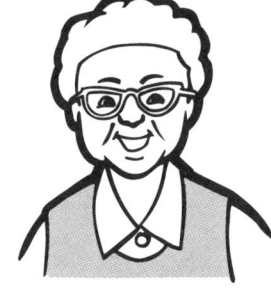
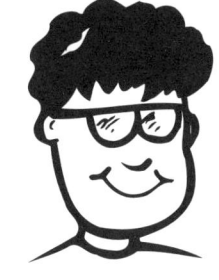
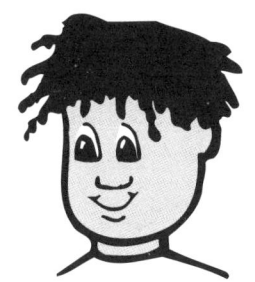

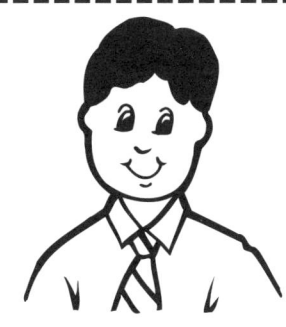
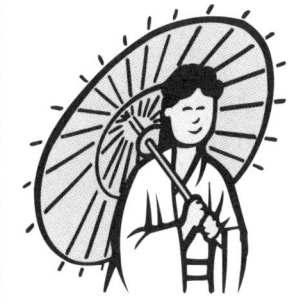
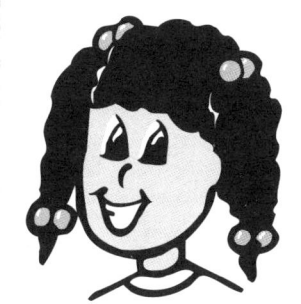

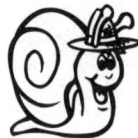 # Farm Pictures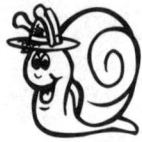

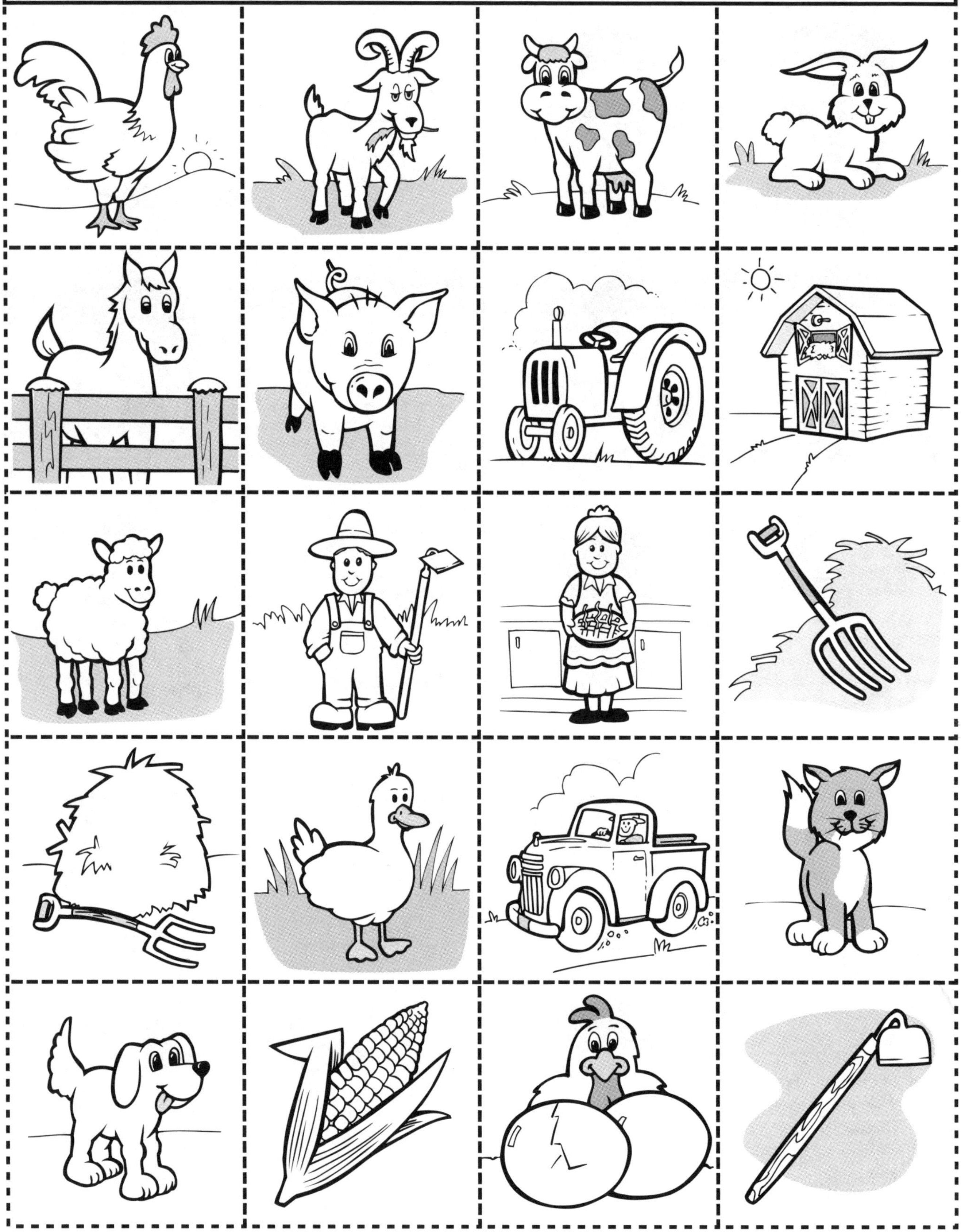

Food

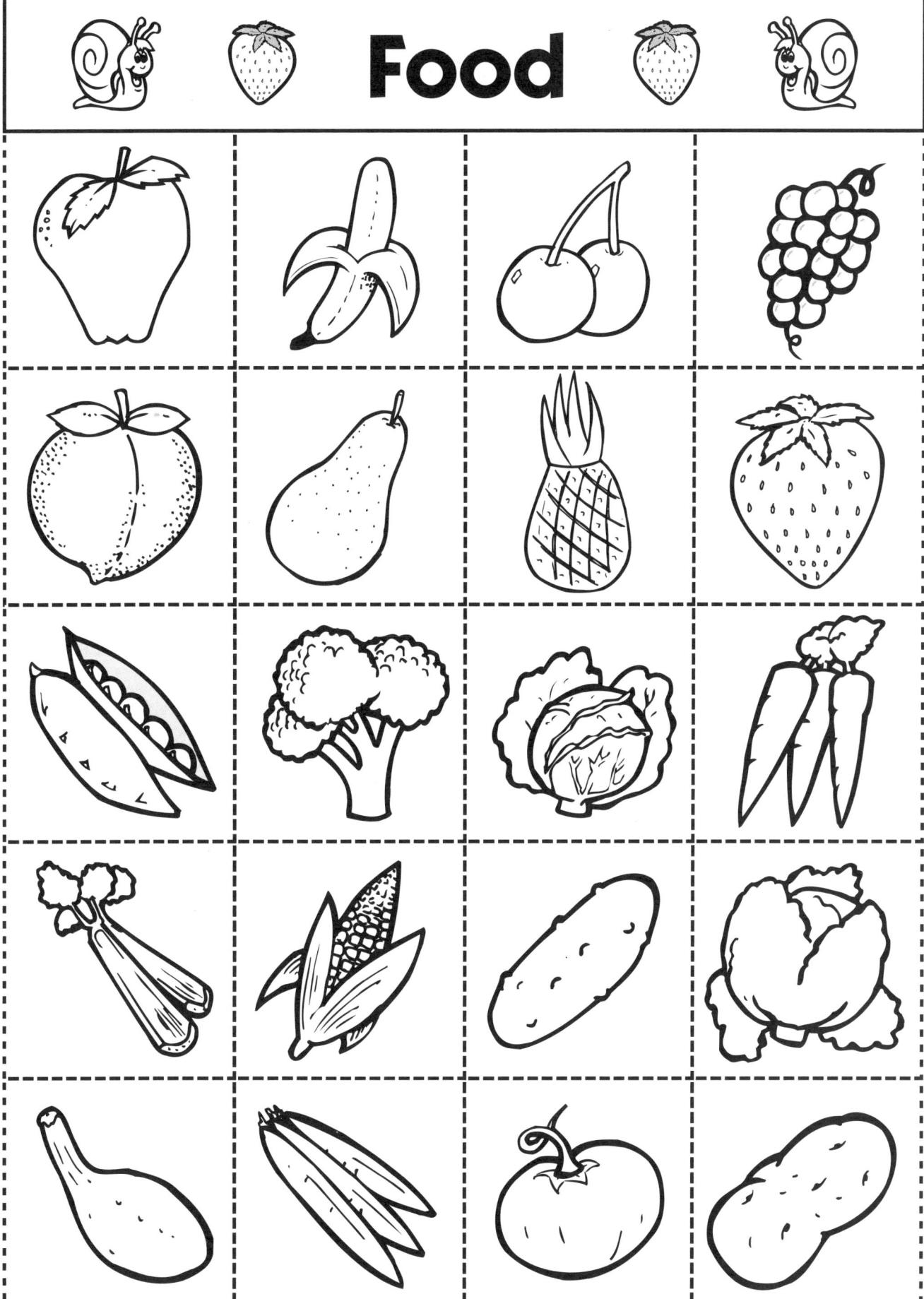

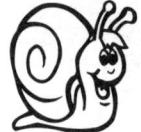 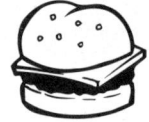 # Food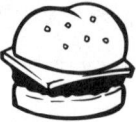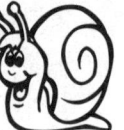

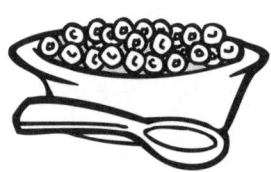   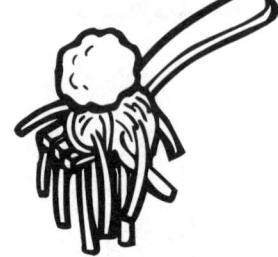

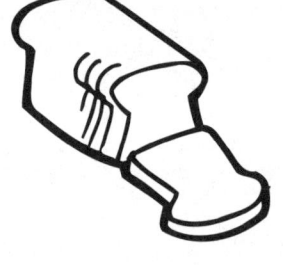  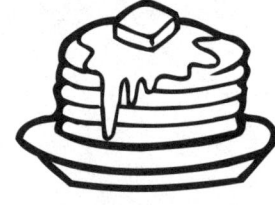 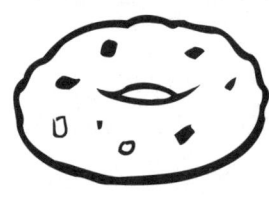

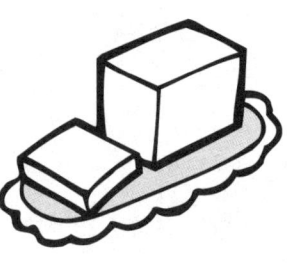 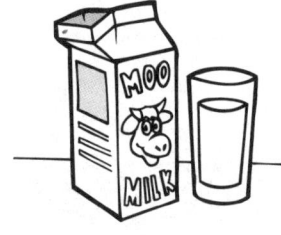 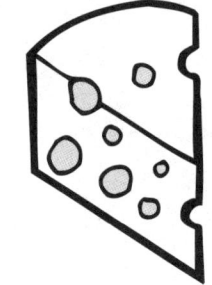 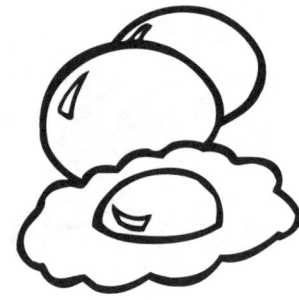

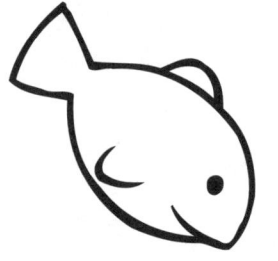 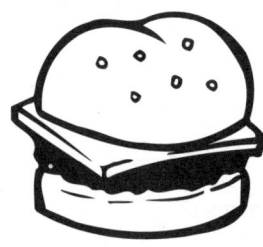 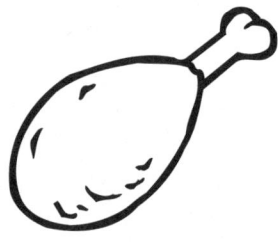 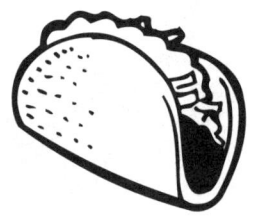

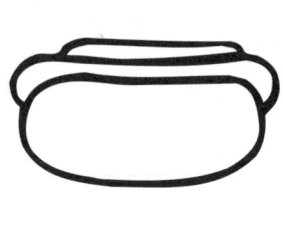 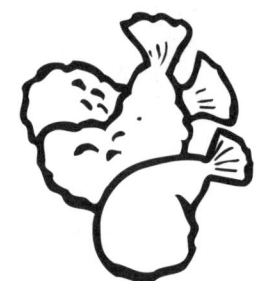 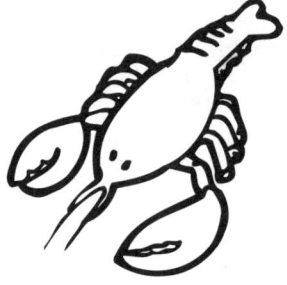 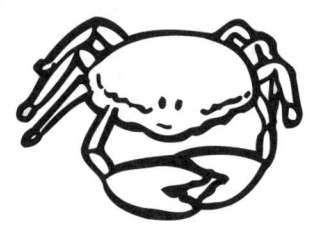

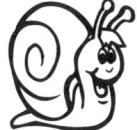 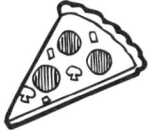 # Food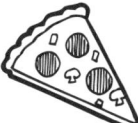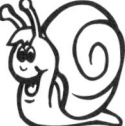

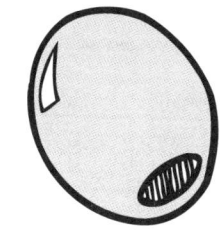 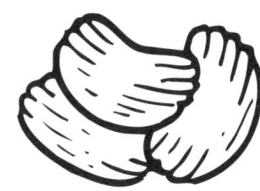 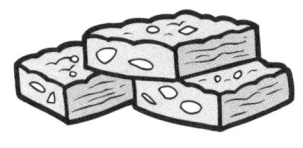 

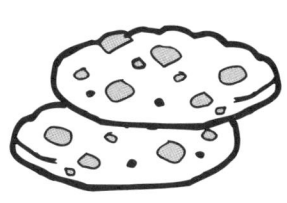 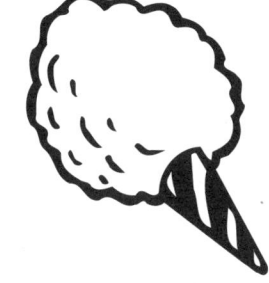  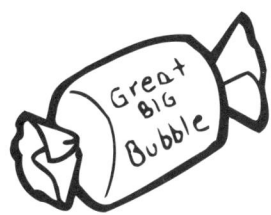

 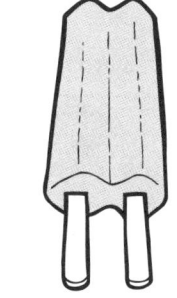 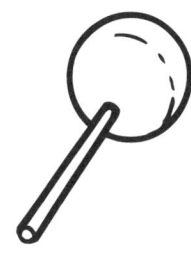 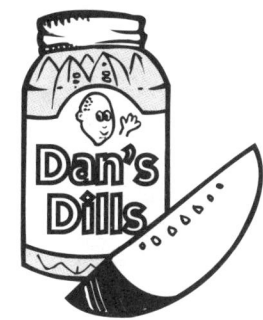

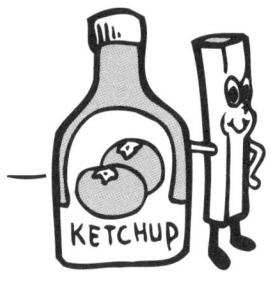 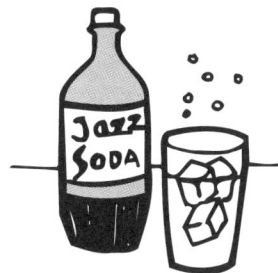 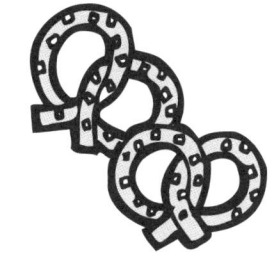 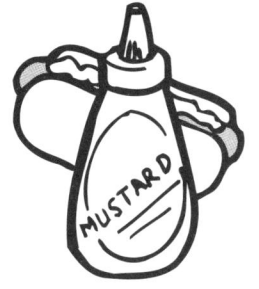

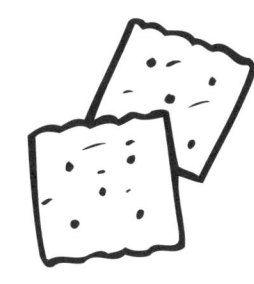  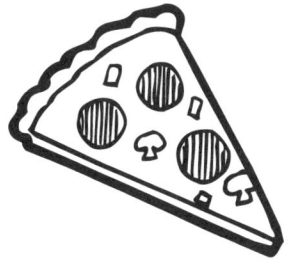 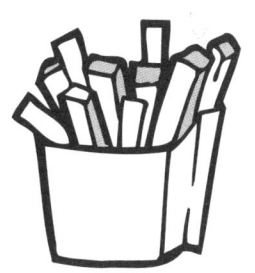

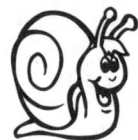 # Grocery Store
(Non-Food Items)
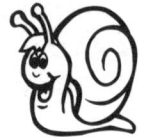

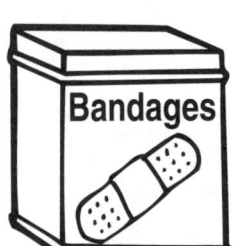  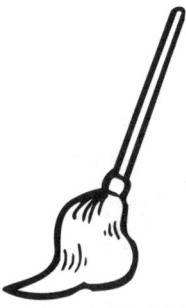 

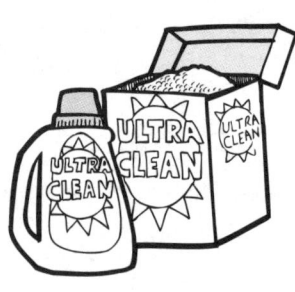 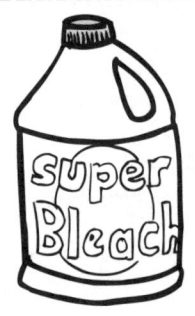 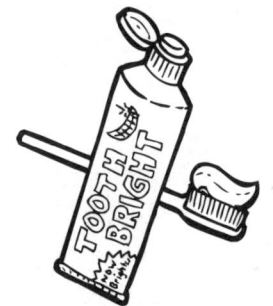 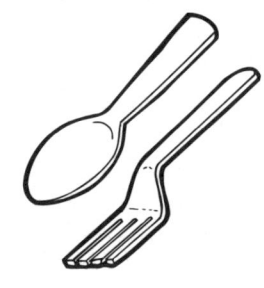

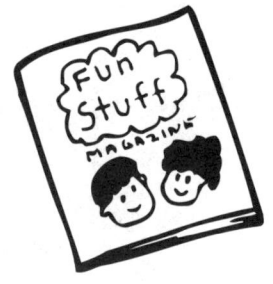 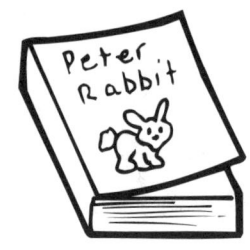 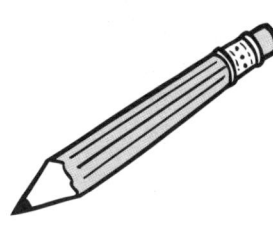 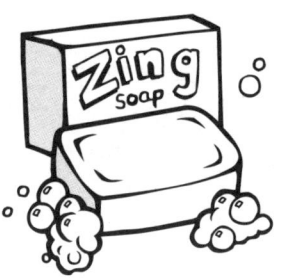

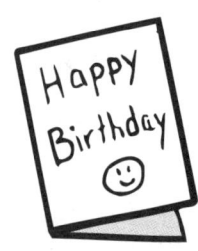 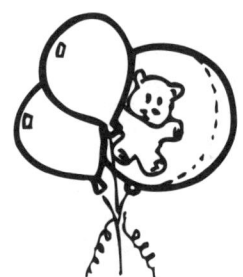 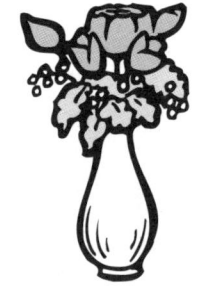 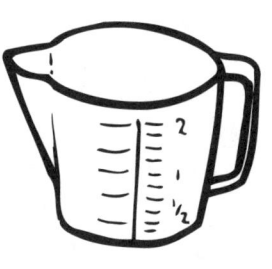

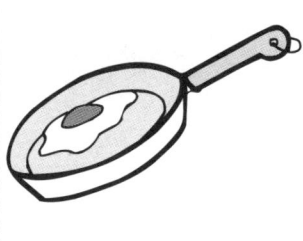 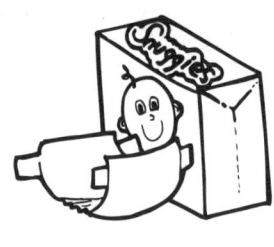 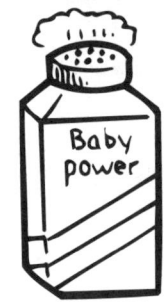 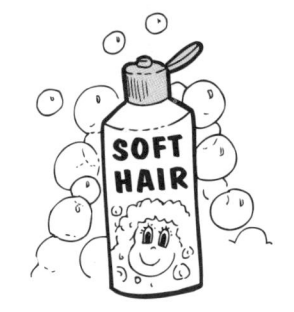

Playground / Toys / Birthday

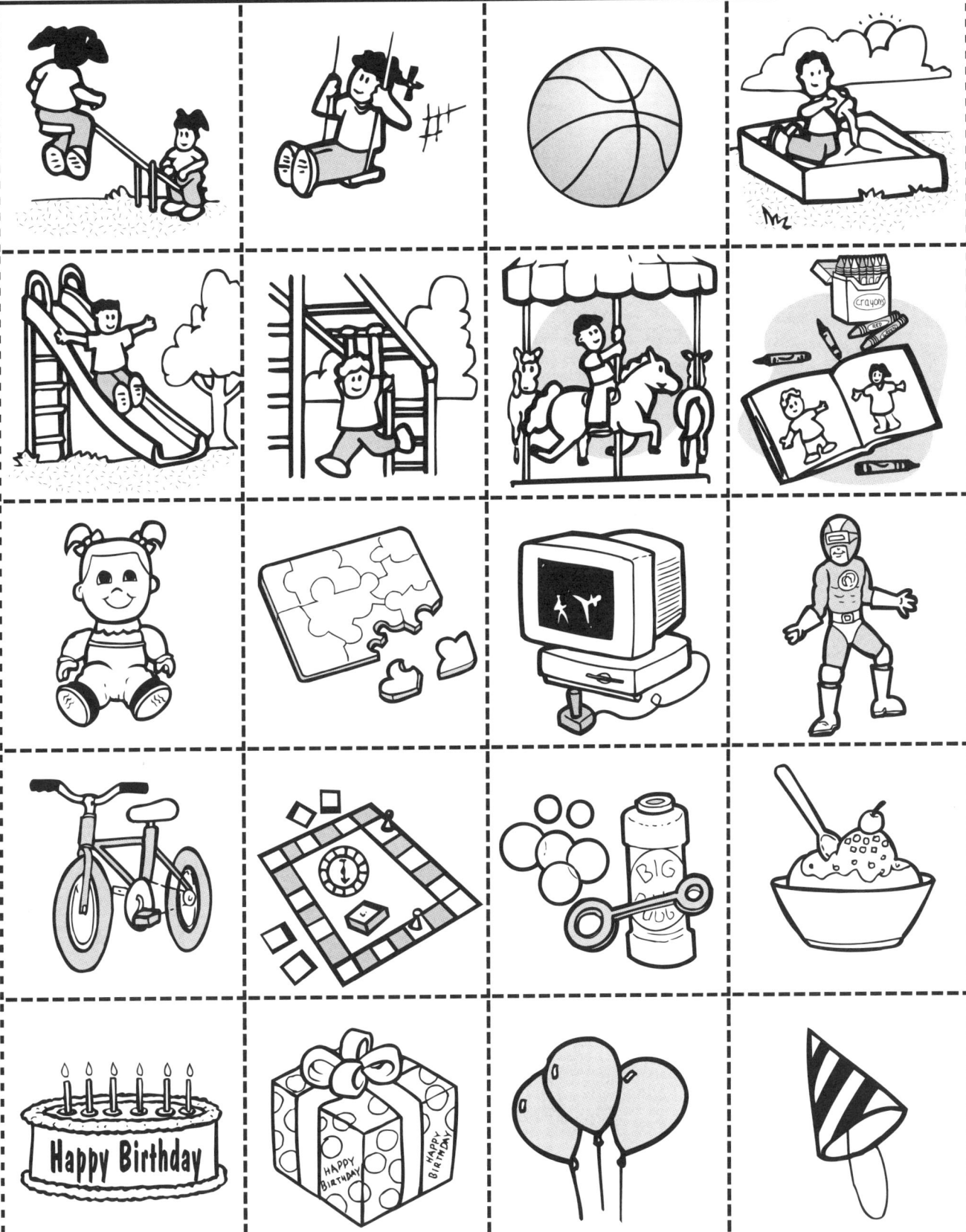

School

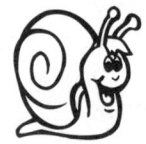 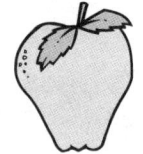 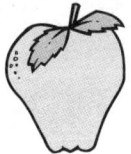 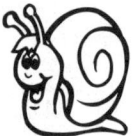

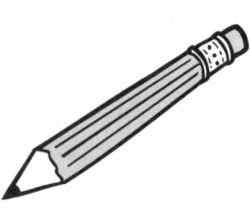 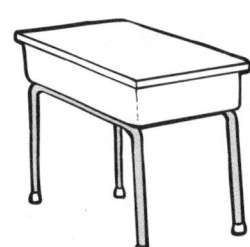 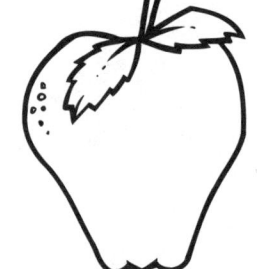 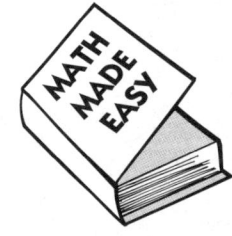

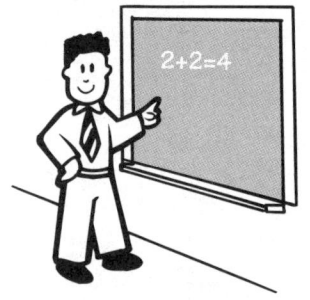 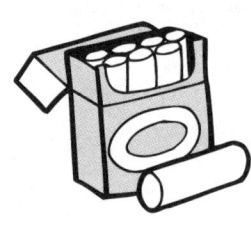 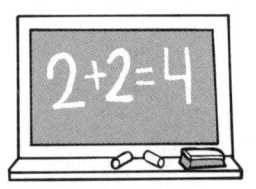 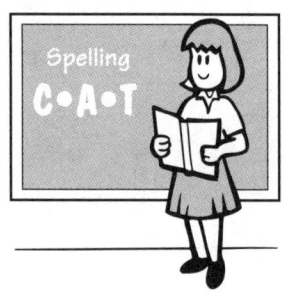

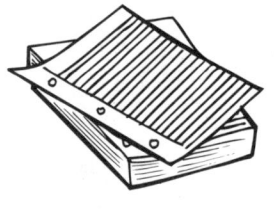 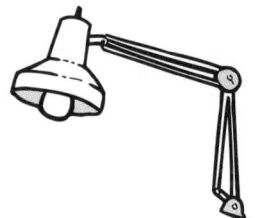 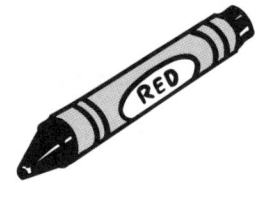 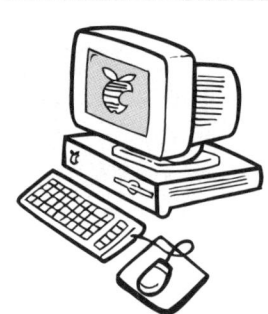

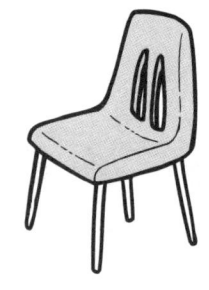  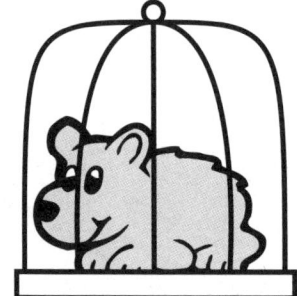 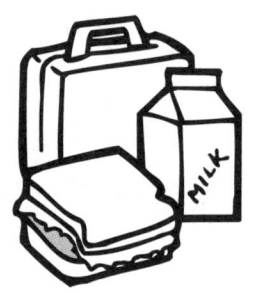

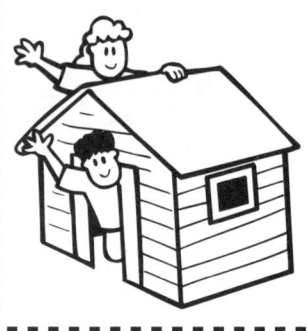 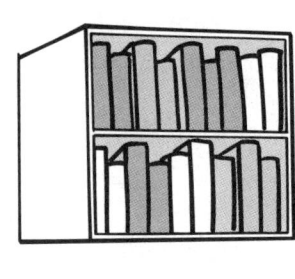 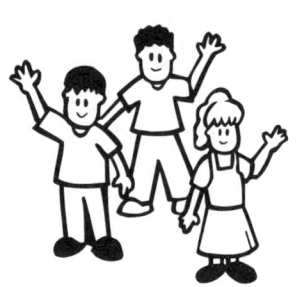 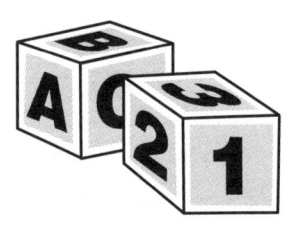

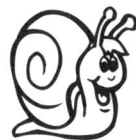 # Things that are Red or Yellow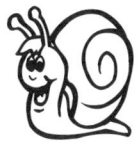

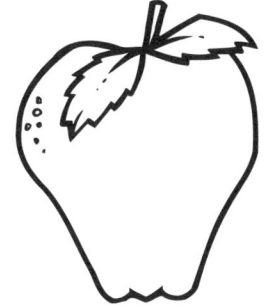 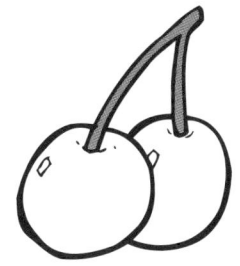 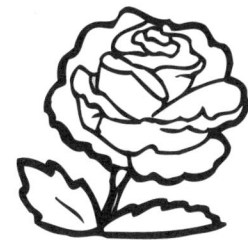 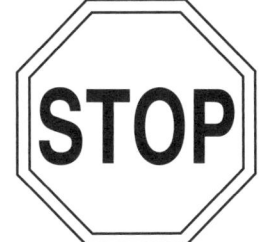

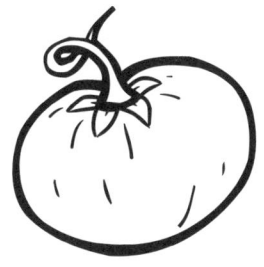 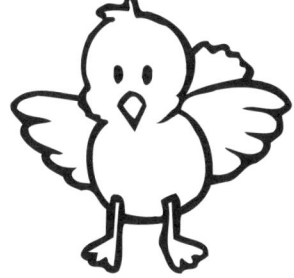 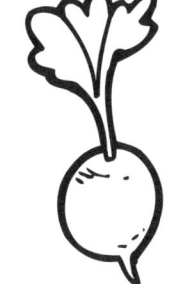 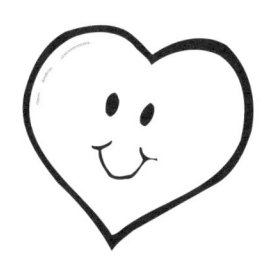

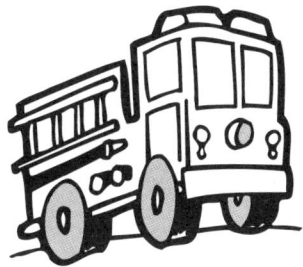 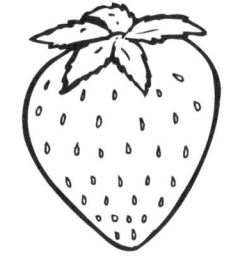 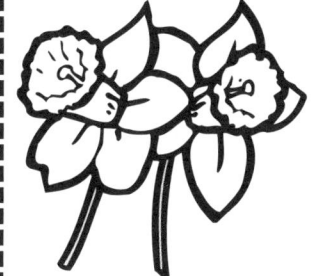 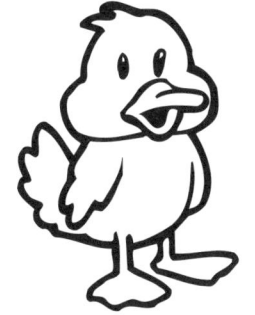

 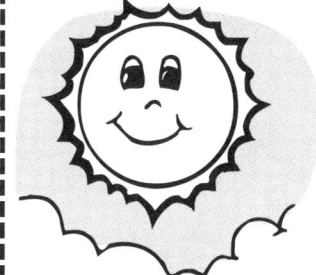 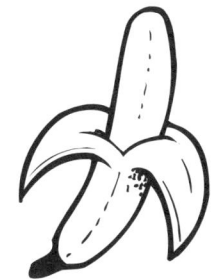 

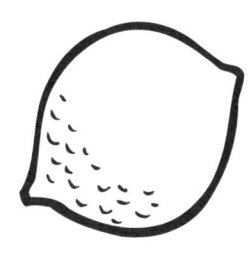 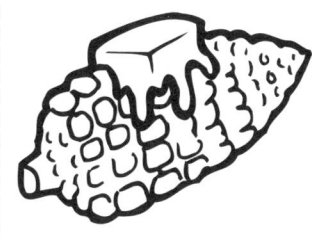 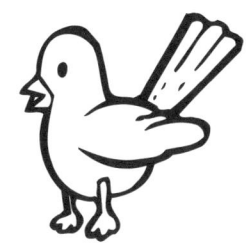 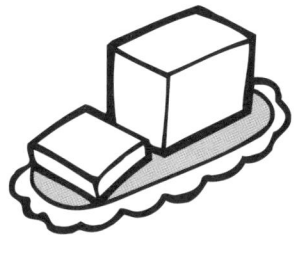

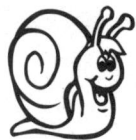 # Zoo Pictures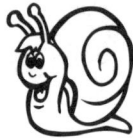

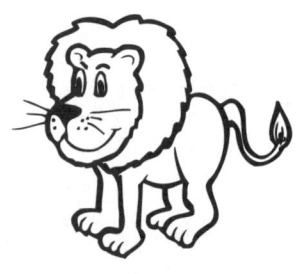 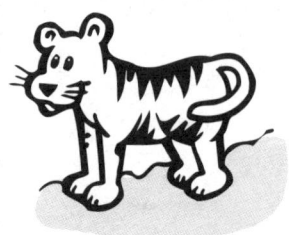 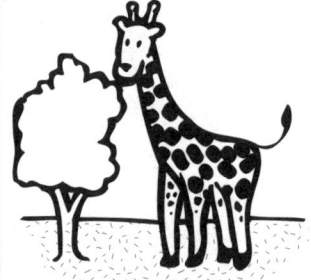 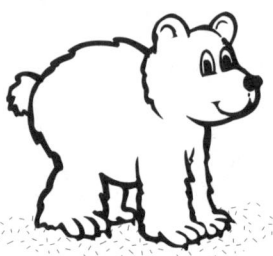

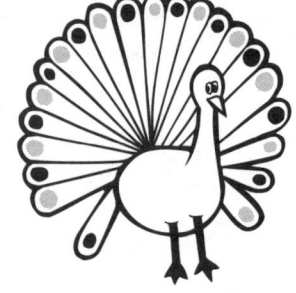 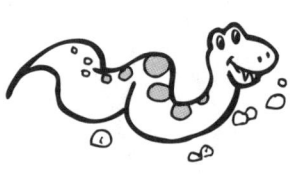 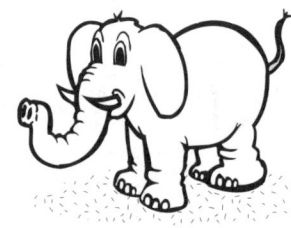 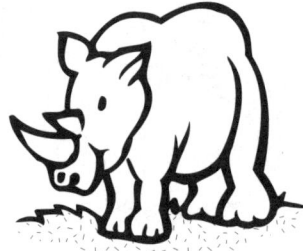

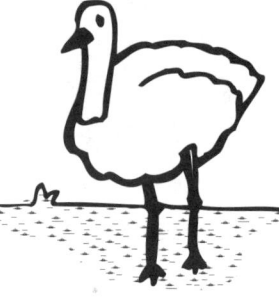 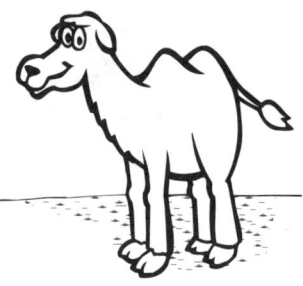 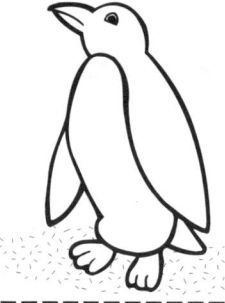 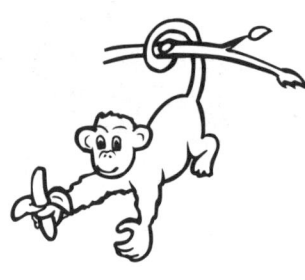

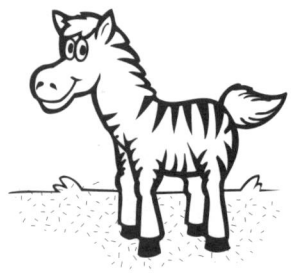  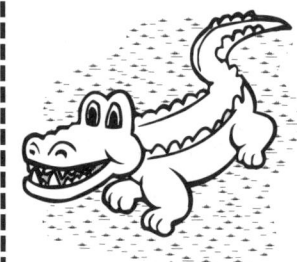 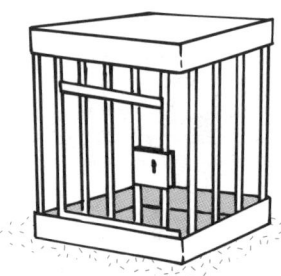

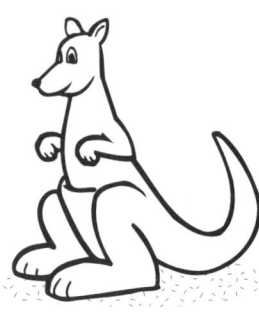 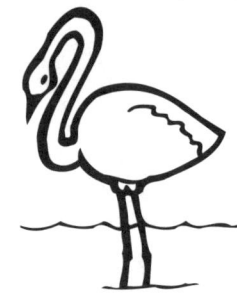 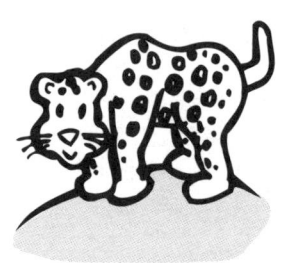 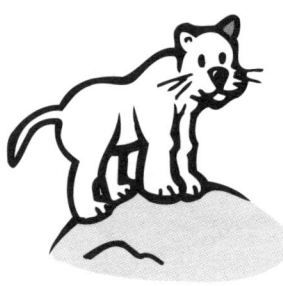

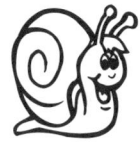 # X-Tra Pictures for Fun!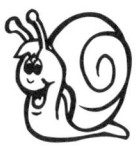

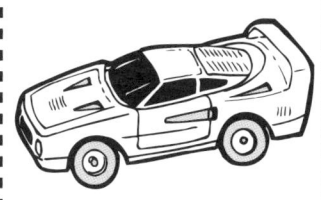 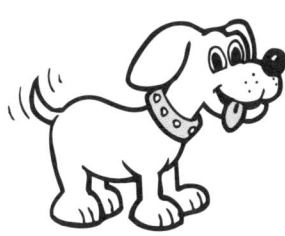 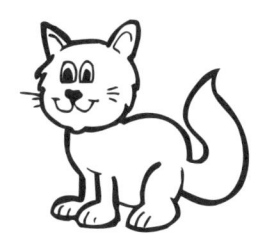 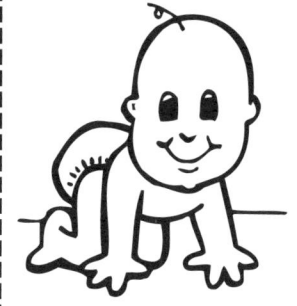

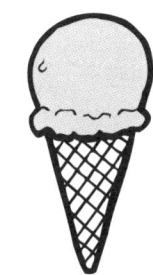 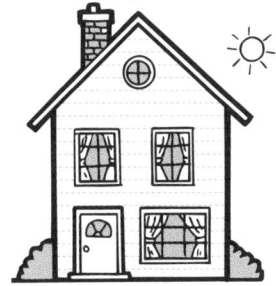 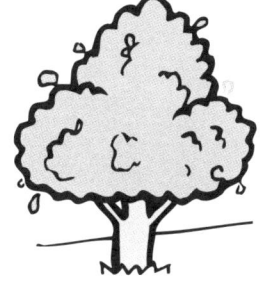 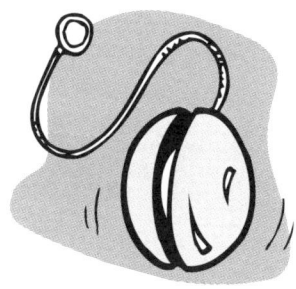

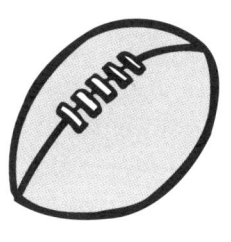 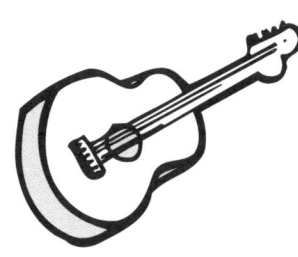 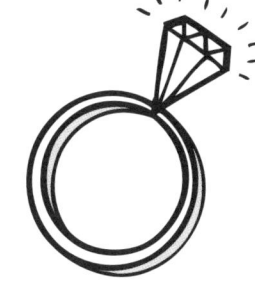 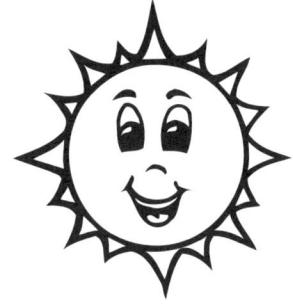

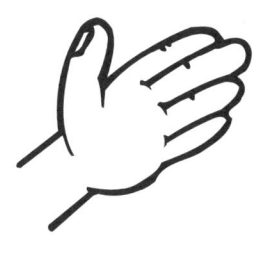 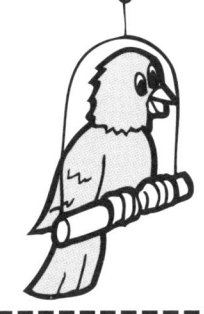 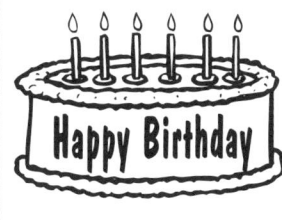 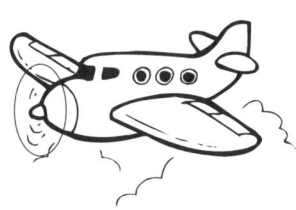

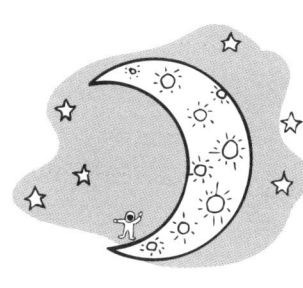 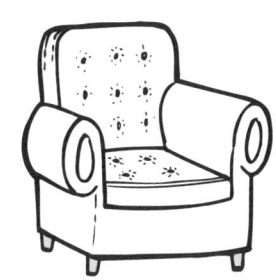 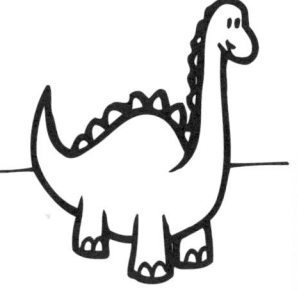 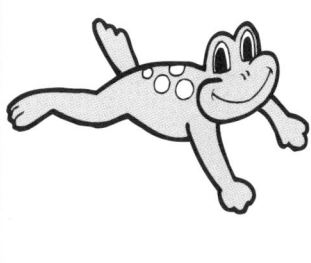

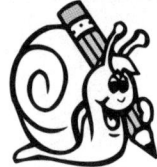
Draw Your Own Pictures!

Notes

Notes

Notes

Notes

Notes

Notes